D0891842

Human poisoning from native and cultivated plants

HUMAN POISONING
FROM NATIVE AND
CULTIVATED PLANTS

James W. Hardin
Jay M. Arena, M.D.

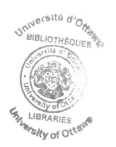

Duke University Press
Durham, North Carolina
1969

© 1969 by Duke University Press
Library of Congress Catalogue Card Number 73-83719
SBN 8223-0209-8

Printed in the United States of America
by Litho Industries, Inc., Raleigh, N. C.

Second printing, 1970

PREFACE

Most of the existing literature on poisonous plants deals with those that are poisonous to livestock. We have felt a real need for a source of information on just those plants poisonous to humans—particularly children. Physicians, health officers, nurses, scout leaders, camp counselors, teachers, parents, and many others should not only know the dangerous plants of their area but have a ready reference in case of emergencies. This book has been written with these people in mind and has grown out of a number of years' experience with poisonous plants accumulated by both of us in the field, laboratory, and clinic.

We are indebted to our colleagues and to the numerous people who have brought cases of human poisoning to our attention and have in various ways contributed to the information presented here. Our information has been combined with details from the literature on poisonous plants, the most complete summary of which is by Dr. John M. Kingsbury of Cornell University, *Poisonous Plants of the United States and Canada* (Prentice-Hall, 1964).

The photographs, unless otherwise credited, were taken by Hardin under a project supported by the North Carolina Agricultural Experiment Station, and many were originally published in that station's Bulletin 414. The support of the research and permission to reproduce the figures are both gratefully acknowledged.

Figures 6–9 were very kindly supplied by Dr. L. R. Hesler, Emeritus Professor of Botany, University of Tennessee; Figures 8 and 9 are from his book *Mushrooms of the Great Smokies,* published by the University of Tennessee Press

(1960) and used here with permission. Figure 18 is from the Missouri Agricultural Experiment Station Bulletin 433 and is used here with permission. Figure 19 was generously supplied by the North Carolina State Bureau of Investigation, and we appreciate the aid of Mr. William S. Best, chemist for the North Carolina SBI, in supplying information on narcotics. Figures or parts of figures 3, 26, 29, 30, 35, 42, 44, 46, and 49 are USDA photographs. The drawings for Figures 5, 15, 24, 47, and 48 are from *Flora of West Virginia* (W. Va. Univ. Bull., 1953, 1958) and are used with the permission of Dr. Earl L. Core. Figures 10, 27, 31, 34, 39, 41, and 45 are from Florida Agricultural Experiment Station Bulletin 510 and Circular S–100. The line drawings, Figures 51–55, are by Hardin, and all but Figure 51 were originally published in his *Workbook for Woody Plants* (Burgess Publishing Company, 1960). We are indeed grateful for all of these illustrations.

JAMES W. HARDIN
JAY M. ARENA

CONTENTS

INTRODUCTION   3

    Thirteen ways to avoid plant poisoning   5

    List of dangerous plants   6

ALLERGIES   9

DERMATITIS   12

    Most common causes of dermatitis   15

    Phytophotodermatitis: Solar dermatitis

       from plants   22

INTERNAL POISONING   25

    First aid: What to do in case of

       internal poisoning   26

    Common Poisonous plants   27

    Poisonous and non-poisonous berries   126

POISONING OF PETS   135

GLOSSARY   137

BIBLIOGRAPHY   148

INDEX TO SCIENTIFIC AND COMMON NAMES   154

ILLUSTRATIONS

1. Common ragweed (*Ambrosia artemisiifolia*)   10
2. Trumpet creeper or cowitch *(Campsis radicans)*   15, 16
3. Poison ivy (*Toxicodendron radicans*)   19, 20
4. Poison sumac (*Toxicodendron vernix*)   21
5. Stinging nettle (*Urtica dioica*)   23
6. Destroying angel (*Amanita verna*)   30
7. Browning amanita (*Amanita brunnescens*)   31
8. Jack-o'-lantern mushroom (*Clitocybe illudens*)   32
9. Morgan's lepiota (*Lepiota molybdites*)   33
10. Glory lily (*Gloriosa superba*)   37
11. Dumbcane (*Dieffenbachia* sp.)   40
12. Jack-in-the-pulpit (*Arisaema triphyllum*)   41
13. Moonseed (*Menispermum canadense*)   43
14. Baneberry (*Actaea pachypoda*)   45
15. Mayapple (*Podophyllum peltatum*)   47
16. Bleeding heart (*Dicentra eximia*)   51
17. Pokeweed (*Phytolacca americana*)   52, 53
18. Corn cockle (*Agrostemma githago*)   55
19. Peyote (*Lophophora williamsii*)   57
20. Black cherry (*Prunus serotina*)   61
21. Jequirity pea or rosary pea (*Abrus precatorius*)   62
22. Black locust (*Robinia pseudoacacia*)   67
23. Wisteria (*Wisteria sinensis*)   69
24. Marijuana (*Cannabis sativa*)   71
25. Virginia creeper (*Parthenocissus quinquefolia*)   76
26. Mistletoe (*Phoradendron serotinum*)   77

27. Chinaberry (*Melia azedarach*)   78
28. Painted buckeye (*Aesculus sylvatica*)   80, 81
29. Water hemlock (*Cicuta maculata*)   84, 85
30. Poison hemlock (*Conium maculatum*)   86, 87
31. Tung nut (*Aleurites fordii*)   89
32. Crown-of-thorns (*Euphorbia milii*)   91
33. Milk bush or pencil tree (*Euphorbia tirucallii*)   93
34. Purge nut or Barbados nut (*Jatropha curcas*)   95
35. Castor bean (*Ricinus communis*)   96, 97
36. Mountain laurel (*Kalmia latifolia*)   99
37. Rhododendron (*Rhododendron maximum*)   101
38. Yellow jessamine (*Gelsemium sempervirens*)   103
39. Yellow allamanda (*Allamanda cathartica*)   104
40. Dogbane (*Apocynum cannabinum*)   105
41. Crape jasmine (*Ervatamia coronaria*)   106
42. Oleander (*Nerium oleander*)   107
43. Elderberry (*Sambucus canadensis*)   110
44. Jimsonweed (*Datura stramonium*)   112
45. Angel's trumpet (*Datura suaveolens*)   115
46. Black nightshade (*Solanum americanum*)   118
47. Horse nettle (*Solanum carolinense*)   119
48. Deadly nightshade (*Solanum dulcamara*)   119
49. Lantana (*Lantana camara*)   123
50. White snakeroot (*Eupatorium rugosum*)   125
51. Parts of a mushroom   140
52. Twigs and leaves   141
53. Leaf forms   142
54. Leaf shapes   143, 144, 145
55. Flower parts and inflorescences   146, 147

Human poisoning from native and cultivated plants

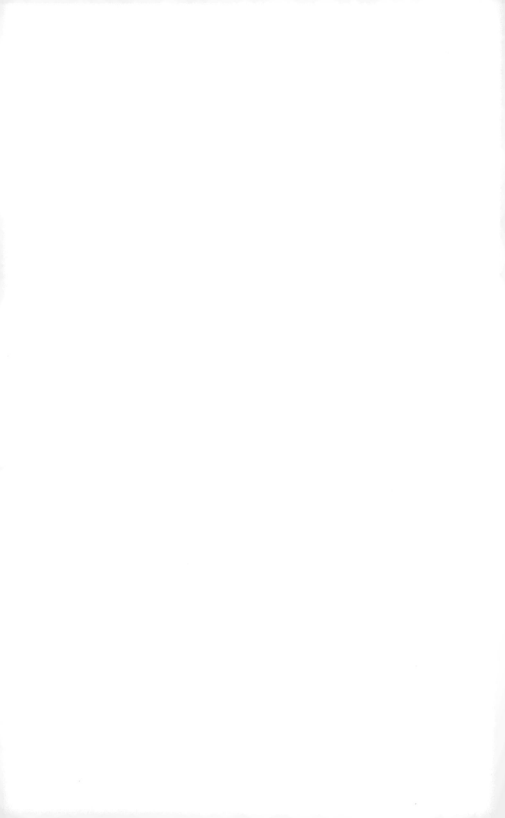

INTRODUCTION

Plants can be dangerous!

Our pioneer forefathers and the agrarian society in general before and through the early nineteenth century had a serious problem with the numerous poisonous plants, few of which were known to them as poisonous. Many of the poisonings reaching near epidemic proportions in those times—such as the "milk sickness" in the Appalachians and Midwest caused by white snakeroot—have been virtually eliminated today by modern food processing and by the fact that a smaller percentage of our population lives in such direct contact with natural vegetation. One might assume from this that plant poisoning to man is no longer a problem. This is not the case, for many areas of North America are still largely rural. Even though there is a constant migration to the cities, there is also a distinct countermigration from the cities into a suburban environment with space for large lawns, gardens, and patios. Suburban plantings are using more and more cultivated exotics from around the world. Increasing numbers of families are camping and hiking in fields and forests and in general are spending more recreation time out-of-doors with plants unfamiliar to them. All these conditions mean that poisonous plants still can be, and still are, the cause of serious illnesses or even death among children and adults. In recent years approximately 3.5 per cent of all poisonings has been due to plants.

In our modern civilization, and particularly in view of our eagerness to return to nature, we should remember that we are seldom out of easy reach of some poisonous plant—whether it be in field or forest, swamp or bog, flower garden or vegetable garden, around the home or in it (see the lists of dangerous plants, pp. 6–8). Poisonous plants are to be found among all types of native plants: algae, fungi, ferns, herbs, vines, shrubs, and trees. Some of our most prized cultivated ornamentals are extremely dangerous (though one should not overlook the fact that symptoms may be caused by sprays applied to ornamentals rather than by the plants themselves).

The term "poisonous plant" designates many kinds of plants as well as a wide range of poisonous or disturbing effects. These effects may generally be classified as: (1) *allergies,* or allergic reactions to wind-blown spores or pollen; (2) *dermatitis,* or skin irritation caused by direct or indirect contact with a plant; (3) *internal poisoning* caused by eating plant parts; and (4) *mechanical injury* from sharp prickles, spines, or thorns found on many plants. The first three categories are the chief concern of this book and will be discussed further; the fourth category may not be considered "poisoning" in the true sense, but mechanical injury may lead to secondary infections requiring medical attention.

Under normal circumstances no adult would think of touching or eating poisonous plants, yet they are contacted and even eaten accidentally or swallowed thoughtlessly. Many poisonous plants have such an unpleasant taste that it is not likely that any adult would chew on them very long or swallow them. But some poisonous plants are not at all distasteful and may be eaten in enough quantity to cause serious disturbances or even death. Fortunately, relatively large amounts of most plants are necessary to produce serious or fatal poisoning in man.

The situation with regard to children is much more dangerous. Small children have a great curiosity and will often chew on anything within reach. Much smaller amounts of the toxin are needed to cause very severe or fatal results. One or two seeds could cause death. Even youngsters will sample almost anything, especially in play or when there is a dare involved.

The objectives of this book are to increase the awareness of these potential dangers, to aid in the identification of the more common poisonous plants native to or cultivated in the United States (including Alaska and Hawaii) and Canada, and to assist physicians in the recognition of symptoms and treatment of such cases.

We do not wish to recommend the elimination or eradication of native and exotic plants which are dangerous, and by no means do we want to make people afraid to venture out-of-doors. All dangers cannot be removed from our surroundings, but we can learn to recognize and avoid them. We do wish, however, to call attention to poisonous plants as potential hazards that surround us so that appropriate precautions can be taken.

We hope that an awareness of these potential dangers, with appropriate education of children, can measurably decrease the number of cases of plant poisoning that occur each year. Plants known to be dangerous should be given the same respect as other, more publicized, household hazards. There is little excuse for the fact that most plant poisonings occur in the home or yard.

Thirteen ways to avoid plant poisoning

1. Become familiar with the dangerous plants in your area, yard, and home. Know them by name.
2. Do not eat wild plants, including mushrooms, unless *positive* of identification.
3. Keep plants, seeds, fruits, and bulbs away from infants.
4. Teach children at an early age to keep unknown plants and plant parts out of their mouths. Make them aware of the potential danger of poisonous plants.
5. Teach children to recognize poison ivy or other causes of dermatitis in your area.
6. Be certain you know the plants used by children as playthings (seeds or fruits, stems, etc.) or as skewers for meat or marshmallows.
7. Do not allow children to suck nectar from flowers or make "tea" from leaves.
8. Know the plant before eating its fruits.
9. Do not rely on pets, birds, or squirrels to indicate non-poisonous plants.

10. Avoid smoke from burning plants, unless you know exactly what they are.

11. Remember, heating and cooking do not always destroy the toxic substance.

12. Store labeled bulbs and seeds safely away from children and pets.

13. Do not make homemade medicines from native or cultivated plants.

List of dangerous plants

Native or naturalized plants of woods, fields, bogs, lawns, and disturbed areas

Dermatitis

Manchineel	Poisonwood	Trumpet creeper
Poison ivy	Spotted spurge	Wild parsnip
Poison oak	Spurge nettle	Woodnettle
Poison sumac	Stinging nettle	

Internal poisons

Apple-of-Peru	Elderberry	Mistletoe
Baneberry	Elephant ear	Monkshood
Beech	False hellebore	Moonseed
Black cherry	Golden seal	Mountain laurel
Black locust	Ground cherry	Mulberry
Black snakeroot	Holly	Mushrooms
Bloodroot	Horse nettle	Nightshade
Blue cohosh	Hydrangea	Oak (acorns)
Buckeye	Jack-in-the-pulpit	Poison hemlock
Buckthorn	Jequirity pea	Pokeweed
Burning bush	Jimsonweed	Prickly poppy
Buttercup	Kentucky coffee	Rattlebox
Chinaberry	tree	Rayless goldenrod
Coontie	Larkspur	Rhododendron
Corn cockle	Lobelia	Rock poppy
Coyotillo	Mayapple	Spurge
Cycads	Mescal bean	Star-of-Bethlehem
Dicentra	Mexican	Strawberry bush
Dogbane	pricklepoppy	Virginia creeper

| Water hemlock | Wild balsam apple | Yellow nightshade |
| White snakeroot | Yellow jessamine | Yew |

Cultivated plants of the yard and garden

Dermatitis

Gas plant

Internal poisons

Akee	Daphne	Narcissus
Amaryllis	Devil's trumpet	Ochrosia plum
Anemone	Dieffenbachia	Oleander
Angel's trumpet	Duranta	Pencil tree
Arnica	English ivy	Physic nut
Autumn crocus	Fava bean	Poinciana
Azalea	Finger cherry	Pongam
Belladonna	Four-o'clock	Prickly poppy
Betel nut	Foxglove	Privet
Bird-of-paradise	Glory lily	Purge nut
Bittersweet	Golden chain	Rattlebox
Black henbane	Hill gooseberry	Rhododendron
Bleeding heart	Holly	Rhubarb
Boxwood	Horsechestnut	Rubber vine
Burning bush	Hyacinth	Sandbox tree
Caladium	Hyacinth bean	Snow-on-the-
Caper spurge	Hydrangea	mountain
Cassava	Jessamine	Spring adonis
Castor bean	Jerusalem cherry	Spurge
Cestrum	Jetbead	Star-of-Bethlehem
Cherry	Kentucky coffee	Sweet pea
Chinaberry	tree	Tobacco
Christmas rose	Larkspur	Tomato
Clematis	Lantana	Trumpet flower
Coca	Laurel	Tung oil tree
Crape jasmine	Lignum vitae	Wisteria
Crownflower	Lily-of-the-valley	Yellow allamanda
Crown-of-thorns	Mescal bean	Yellow jessamine
Cycads	Monkshood	Yellow oleander
Cypress spurge	Mustard	Yew

House plants

Amaryllis	Dieffenbachia	Narcissus
Bird-of-paradise	Glory lily	Pencil tree
Crown-of-thorns	Hyacinth	Philodendron
		Poinsettia

Christmas greenery

Boxwood	Holly	Mountain laurel
English ivy	Jequirity pea	Poinsettia
European	Jerusalem cherry	Yew
bittersweet	Mistletoe	

Narcotics—Hallucinogenic drugs

Betel nut	Morning glory	Nutmeg
Coca	seeds (heavenly	Opium poppy
Marijuana	blue, pearly	Peyote
	gates)	

ALLERGIES

Allergy is a condition of unusual sensitivity which certain individuals may have or develop to substances ordinarily harmless. These sensitizing substances are called allergens. Spores from numerous fungi, some soil algae, and pollen grains from seed plants cause allergic reactions in susceptible individuals. These wind-blown plant structures (aero-allergens) are "poisonous" in the broad sense. There are estimated to be thirteen million sufferers from plant aero-allergens each year.

Fungi are all around us. The spores are microscopic in size and are easily carried in the atmosphere. The humid areas of North America have a fairly high and constant count of atmospheric fungus spores. Certain microscopic soil algae are also wind-blown and cause allergic reactions.

Pollen counts are more seasonal depending upon the flowering period for certain plant species. There are generally three seasonal peaks in the frequency of pollen in the atmosphere. The first is in the early spring, caused by the early flowering of such trees as oak, elm, cedar (juniper), maple, sycamore, ash, alder, birch, poplar, hickory, beech, and others throughout the country. The counts are highest in the deciduous forest area of the eastern United States and amount to a few hundred pollen grains per cubic yard of atmosphere. The problem of treatment is complicated by the great number of different kinds of trees involved.

The second peak in pollen frequency comes in midsummer and is caused primarily by grasses of various types, some herbs, and a few late-flowering trees. The counts at this time may also be a few hundred grains per cubic yard of atmosphere and are fairly equally distributed throughout the country.

The third and highest peak comes in the fall with the flowering of ragweeds and a few other herbs. Ragweeds (Figure 1) are found throughout the country, and the pollen is by far the most abundant and most toxic of all aero-

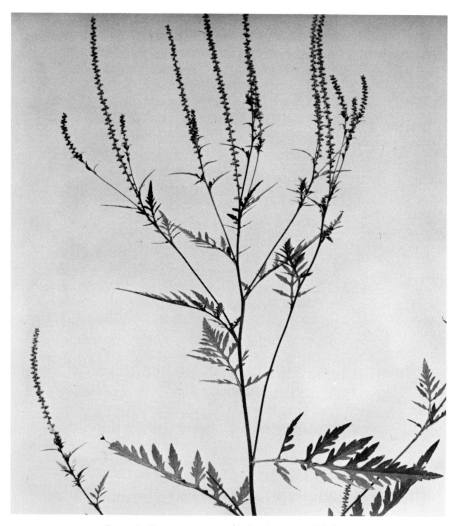

Figure 1. Common ragweed (*Ambrosia artemisiifolia*) A ubiquitous weed with terminal spikes of numerous pollen flowers.

allergens. Ragweed counts range from a few hundred to nearly two thousand grains per cubic yard of atmosphere. Most of the eastern United States has a high count, but in the plains area between the Rockies and the Appalachians the great abundance of ragweed pollen is astonishing. This "breadbasket of America" is a veritable pollen basket as well, for almost every wheat field is also a ragweed field.

There are a few real refuges from ragweed pollen. Very low counts are found in northern Wisconsin, the upper peninsula of Michigan, the mountains of upper New York, Maine, and New Hampshire, central and eastern Canada, southern Florida and the Caribbean, and west of the Rocky Mountains. Alaska and Hawaii have hardly any ragweed pollen.

Hay fever, untreated, may lead to asthma and other serious complications. The asthmatic child, if his particular sensitivity is not detected and if proper care is not given, may be retarded physically and may have permanent involvement of the heart, lungs, and chest wall with invalidism. If allergy is at all suspected, see your physician or allergist as soon as possible

DERMATITIS

There are numerous plants which may cause dermatitis, an irritation to the skin. Any one individual may be susceptible to many of these plants, to only a few, or to none at all. Dermatitis, like allergy, is dependent upon a previous sensitivity of the individual.

The degree of poisoning may vary from minor or temporary skin irritation to very painful inflammation with blisters persisting for weeks and possibly requiring hospitalization. The severity depends on the plant contacted, the degree of contact, and the relative susceptibility of the individual. Those plants considered to be the most troublesome are listed below preceded by an asterisk(*) and are described following this tabulation of all those suspected of causing dermatitis. (The abbreviation spp. means any of the various species rather than a particular one.)

Scientific name	Common name	Plant part
Agave spp.	Century plant	sap
Ailanthus altissima	Tree-of-heaven	leaves, flowers
Allamanda cathartica	Yellow allamanda	all parts
Ambrosia artemisiifolia	Ragweed	leaves
Anacardium occidentale	Cashew nut	nut shell, oil
Anagallis arvensis	Scarlet pimpernel	leaves
Anthemis cotula	Dog fennel	leaves, flowers
Aralia spinosa	Hercules' club	bark
Arisaema triphyllum	Jack-in-the-pulpit	leaves, roots

Asarum canadense	Wild ginger	leaves
Asimina triloba	Pawpaw	fruits
Asparagus officinalis	Asparagus	young stems
Buxus sempervirens	Boxwood	leaves
Campsis radicans	Trumpet creeper, cowitch	leaves, flowers
Capsicum frutescens	Bird pepper	fruit
Carica papaya	Papaya	sap
Caryota mitis	Tufted fishtail palm	fruit
Catalpa spp.	Catalpa	flowers
Caulophyllum thalictroides	Blue cohosh	roots
Chelidonium majus	Celandine	juice
Chimaphila umbellata	Prince's pine, pipsisscwa	leaves, stems
Chrysanthemum spp.	Chrysanthemum, daisy	leaves
Citrus aurantifolia	Lime	thorn, peels
Clematis virginiana	Virgin's bower	leaves
Cnidoscolus spp.	Spurge nettle, stinging spurge	stinging hairs
Conium maculatum	Poison hemlock	leaves
Cryptostegia madagascariensis	Rubber vine	all parts
Cypripedium spp.	Lady's slipper orchid	leaves
Datura stramonium	Jimsonweed	leaves, flowers
Daucus carota	Wild carrot	leaves
Delphinium ajacis	Larkspur	leaves, seeds
Dicentra spp.	Bleeding heart	all parts
Dirca palustris	Leatherwood	bark
Erigeron canadensis	Daisy fleabane, horseweed	leaves
Euphorbia spp.	Spurge, poinsettia, pencil tree	milky juice
Ficus spp.	Fig	juice

Gelsemium sempervirens	Yellow jessamine	leaves, stems
Ginkgo biloba	Ginkgo, maidenhair tree	seeds
Grevillea banksii	Kahili flower	all parts
Hedera helix	English ivy	leaves
*Hesperocnide spp.	Western stinging nettle	stinging hairs
*Hippomane mancinella	Manchineel	milky juice
Hypericum perforatum	St. John's wort	leaves
Iris spp.	Iris, flag	rhizomes
Juniperus virginiana	Juniper, red cedar	leaves
*Laportea canadensis	Wood nettle	stinging hairs
Leonurus cardiaca	Motherwort	leaves
Lobelia inflata	Lobelia, Indian tobacco	leaves
Maclura pomifera	Osage orange, horse apple	milky juice
Mangifera indica	Mango	sap, fruit peel
Melaleuca leucadenra	Punk tree, cajeput	sap
*Metopium toxiferum	Poisonwood	all parts
Morus rubra	Red mulberry	leaves, stem
Nerium oleander	Oleander	leaves
Phacelia spp.	Phacelia	leaves
Pithecellobium dulce	Pithecellobium	sap
Plumbago capensis	Plumbago	all parts
Plumeria spp.	Frangipani	sap
Podophyllum peltatum	Mayapple, mandrake	roots
Polygonum spp.	Smartweed, knotweed	leaves
Polyscias spp.	Polyscias	all parts
Primula spp.	Primrose	leaves
Ranunculus spp.	Buttercup	leaves
Rhaphidophora aurea	Hunter's robe	sap

Rhoeo spathacea	Oyster plant	sap
Rumex spp.	Dock, sorrel	leaves
Sanguinaria canadensis	Bloodroot	sap
Schinus terebinthifolius	Brazilian pepper	flowers, fruits
Senecio confusus	Mexican flame vine	all parts
Setcreasea purpurea	Purple queen	sap
Toxicodendron spp.	Poison oak, ivy and sumac	all parts
Trifolium hybridum	Alsike clover	leaves
Urtica dioica	Stinging nettle	stinging hairs
Veratrum spp.	Hellebore	leaves

Most common causes of dermatitis

Campsis radicans (L.) Seeman—Trumpet creeper, cowitch (Figure 2)

Description: Woody vine, climbing along fences or high in shrubs, trees, and poles; leaves opposite, pinnately divided into 9-11 ovate leaflets with toothed margins; flowers in

Figure 2. Trumpet creeper or cowitch (*Campsis radicans*) A common vine of eastern United States with divided leaves, yellow to red tubular flowers, and pod-like fruits with many winged seeds. (See next page.)

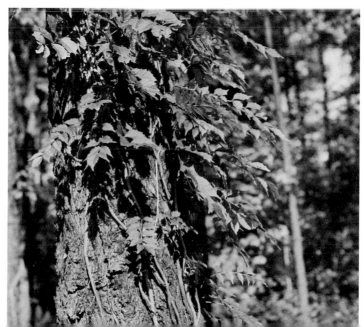

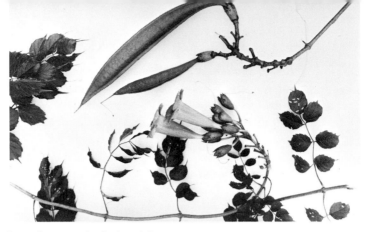

clusters, tubular, 5-lobed, orange-yellow to red, 2–3 in. long; fruit an elongated slender capsule with many winged seeds.

Occurrence: Trumpet creeper grows in moist or dry woods, along fence rows, on roadsides, and in thickets. It is a native vine throughout eastern United States.

Poisoning: Contact with leaves or flowers may cause inflammation of the skin with blisters persisting for a few days.

Cnidoscolus stimulosus (Michx.) Engelm. & Gray (*Jatropha stimulosa* Michx.)—Spurge nettle, stinging spurge, bull nettle, tread-softly

Description: A perennial herb with a short, stout stem and very deep taproot; plant covered with bristly hairs 2–6 mm. long; leaves alternate, palmately veined, rounded, and deeply 3–5-lobed; flowers white, 5-parted, and showy.

Occurrence: Spurge nettle is native and common in sandy woods, fields, or roadsides of the eastern Coastal Plain and Piedmont from Virginia to Florida and west to Texas. Related species are found in south central and southwestern United States.

Poisoning: The stinging hairs, found abundantly on leaves and stems, contain a caustic irritant causing painful inflammation and itching or very severe reaction upon contact. Fainting has been reported in the most severe cases. The structure of the hair is similar to that in *Laportea*.

Euphorbia maculata L.—Spotted spurge, eyebane, milk purslane, wartweed

> Description: Herbaceous perennial with milky juice; stem erect or prostrate; leaves opposite, dark green, and usually with a dark reddish spot near the middle, hairy, oblong, to ¾ in. long, margin with very small teeth; "flowers" small and inconspicuous with minute white bracts.
>
> Occurrence: Eyebane is a native herb throughout eastern and midwestern United States and is an occasional weed in the Pacific states. It grows as a weed in lawns, gardens, waste places, roadsides, and fields. Other species of *Euphorbia,* including poinsettia, found in all parts of the country or cultivated, may be equally poisonous to some people.
>
> Poisoning: Inflammation developing after contact and forming large blisters lasting several days. Small children seem most susceptible.

Hippomane mancinella L.—Manchineel

> Description: Tree to 50 ft. tall with milky juice; leaves alternate, simple, long stalked, the blades broadly ovate to elliptical, 2–6 in. long, margin finely toothed; flowers small, greenish, in stiff spikes; fruit a drupe about 1½ in. across.
>
> Occurrence: Manchineel is a native tree found originally in hammocks near the coast at the southern tip of Florida and on the Keys. It is now rare except in the Everglades National Park.
>
> Poisoning: Severe skin reaction and temporary blindness if eyes are rubbed with infected fingers. This has the reputation of being one of the worst causes of dermatitis in the country. The milky juice was once used by Indians as a poison for arrow tips and also as an ingredient for native medicines.

Laportea canadensis (L.) Wedd.—Wood nettle, nettle

> Description: Erect perennial herb to 5 ft. tall and with conspicuous stinging hairs throughout; leaves alternate, stalked, broadly ovate to 6 in. long, pointed at apex, coarsely toothed; flowers small and inconspicuous, in slender branches from the leaf axils.

Occurrence: Wood nettle is native in various areas throughout eastern United States. It is usually found in moist woods and along streams or rivers, roadsides, and ditches, often forming dense local populations.

Poisoning: Intense burning and itching or stinging of the skin persisting for various lengths of time. The stinging hairs have a mechanism similar to a hypodermic. There is a very fine capillary tube, a bladder-like base filled with the chemical irritant, and a minute spherical tip which easily breaks off on contact, leaving a very sharp-pointed tip which easily penetrates the skin. The chemical is forced into the skin through the tube as the hair bends and constricts the bladder-like base. The irritating chemicals are histamine, acetylcholine, and 5-hydroxytryptamine (5-HT), rather than formic acid as once thought. The stinging hairs of *Cnidoscolus, Hesperocnide,* and *Urtica* are of similar structure.

Metopium toxiferum (L.) Krug & Urban—Poisonwood, coral sumac

Description: Shrub or tree to 35 ft. tall; leaves alternate, pinnately divided with 3–7 (usually 5) leaflets, each leathery and to 3½ in. long; flowers yellow-green, in panicles; fruit oval, to ½ in. across, orange-yellow.

Occurrence: Poisonwood is a native tree of hammocks, pinelands, and along the coast at the southern tip of Florida and on the Keys.

Poisoning: The sap causes very severe skin irritation similar to poison ivy, appearing a few hours to 5 days after contact. Fever and other internal complications can result in very severe cases.

Toxicodendron diversilobum (T. & G.) Green (*Rhus diversiloba* T. & G.)—Western poison oak

This species is similar to poison ivy and is found commonly from British Columbia southward into Mexico. It grows in low places, thickets, and wooded slopes usually below 5,000 ft. elevation.

Poisoning: See *T. vernix.*

Toxicodendron quercifolium (Michx.) Greene (*Rhus toxicodendron* L.)—Poison oak

Description: Shrub, never climbing; leaves alternate, with 3 leaflets, each densely hairy below, deeply toothed or lobed, and coarse-looking; flowers and fruits in hanging clusters, the fruit a yellowish and hairy drupe.

Occurrence: A native shrub, poison oak is more or less restricted to sandy soil, dry barrens, sand hills, oak-pine or pine woods, in New Jersey, Maryland, Tennessee, and southern Missouri south to northern Florida, Texas, and Kansas. It is not as common as poison ivy.

Poisoning: See *T. vernix.*

Toxicodendron radicans (L.) Kuntze (*Rhus radicans* L.)—Poison ivy (Figure 3)

Description: Either a non-climbing woody shrub or a vine climbing along the ground, on low plants, or high in trees or on poles; leaves alternate, with three leaflets, each hairless

Figure 3. Poison ivy (*Toxicodendron radicans*) The infamous weed of the United States and Canada with the characteristic three leaflets. (See next page.)

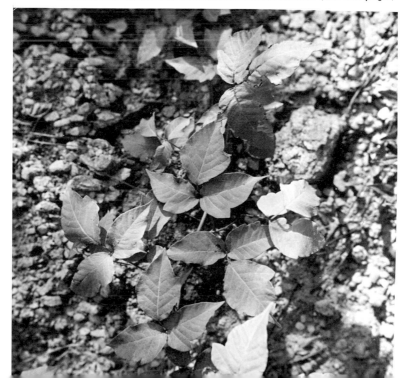

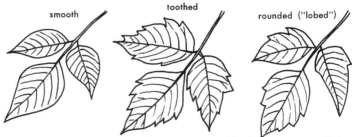

smooth   toothed   rounded ("lobed")

Figure 3, continued. Outlines (USDA Photograph) show variation of the leaflet margin; the lobed form is similar to poison oak.

or slightly hairy, the margin not toothed, with small teeth or variously lobed; flowers and fruits in hanging clusters, the fruit a yellowish drupe, not hairy.

Occurrence: Poison ivy is a native and extremely variable weed throughout southern Canada and the United States except the west coast. It is very common in disturbed places, on flood plains, along lake shores, edges of woods, stream banks, fences, and around buildings.

Poisoning: See *T. vernix*.

Toxicodendron vernix (L.) Kuntze (*Rhus vernix* L.)—Poison sumac, poison elder, poison ash, swamp sumac, thunderwood (Figure 4)

Description: Shrub 5–8 ft. tall, or a small tree to 25 ft. tall, with smooth light gray bark; leaves alternate, pinnately divided with 7–11 leaflets, leaf and leaflet stalks reddish; leaflets pointed, margin not toothed; fruits in hanging clusters, each a cream-yellow, hairless drupe.

Occurrence: Poison sumac is a native in bogs of the North (a shrub) and swamps and river bottoms of the South (a small tree). It is rare in the mountains and most common in the Great Lakes region and eastern Coastal Plain from New Hampshire to Florida and west to Texas.

Poisoning: Every year nearly two million people in the United States experience irritating or painful effects from direct or indirect contact with poison oak, poison ivy, or poison sumac. One out of every two persons is allergic in some degree.

The skin irritant is present in the sap, which is found in the roots, stems, leaves, pollen, flowers, and fruits. The itchy or painful skin rash results from contact with the sap that is released by a bruised portion of the plant. The danger of poisoning is greatest in spring and summer when the sap is abundantly produced and the plant easily bruised.

In addition to direct contact with the plants, the irritant may be spread by dogs, cats, or other animals; by contaminated clothing, garden or yard tools, or sports equipment such as golf clubs, guns, or fishing rods; or by accidental eating of the fruits. The irritating chemical is not volatile, but droplets may be carried in smoke on dust particles or ash. It is therefore dangerous to be in the smoke from burning plants. The pollen is blown by wind, and it is possible for an extremely susceptible person to contact the poison merely by being near the plant when the pollen is in the air.

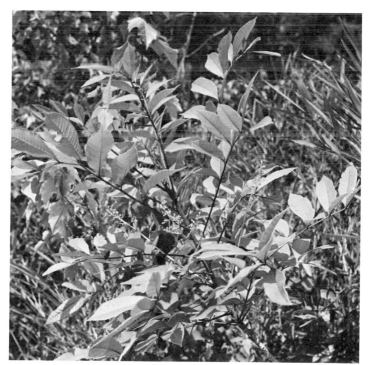

Figure 4. Poison sumac (*Toxicodendron vernix*) A poisonous shrub of bogs and swamps.

After contact, the first symptoms of itching, burning, redness, and small blisters may appear in a matter of a few hours or may take as many as 5 days, depending on the individual. Severe dermatitis, with large blisters and local swelling may remain for several days and may require hospitalization. Persistent symptoms and apparent spreading are generally due to new contacts with plants or previously contaminated objects, or possibly by spread of the irritant from scratched affected skin areas and broken blisters. Secondary infections may occur when blisters are broken.

Proper identification and knowledge of the plants are essential in prevention. Eradication by means of digging or through chemical herbicides (2,4-D; 2,4,5-T; amitrole; ammonium sulfamate) is the most effective means of eliminating repeated contact with plants around the home.

In case of contact, *immediate* washing with strong soap will often prevent the symptoms. If severe symptoms occur, see your physician.

Urtica dioica L.—Stinging nettle (Figure 5)

Description: Erect perennial herb similar to *Laportea* except for opposite leaves.

Occurrence: Stinging nettle grows along roadsides, in moist woods, and in waste places. It is nearly cosmopolitan either as a native or introduced weed. Related species of *Laportea* and also *Hesperocnide* are found in various areas of the United States and Hawaii.

Poisoning: The structure of the stinging hairs and the chemical irritants are the same as in *Laportea*.

Phytophotodermatitis: Solar dermatitis from plants

Numerous plants of wide distribution are thought to cause dermatitis by a combination of sunlight and contact with the plant, but proven photosensitization is rare. Two plants which contain furocoumarins and are known to cause phytophotodermatitis readily are the wild parsnip (*Pastinaca sativa* L.) and dittany or gas plant (*Dictamnus albus* L.).

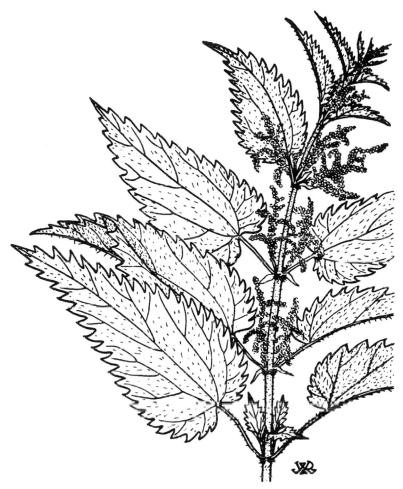

Figure 5. Stinging nettle (*Urtica dioica*) A weedy herb with flower clusters in the axils of opposite leaves and stinging hairs on the stem. From *Flora of West Virginia*, courtesy of Dr. E. L. Core.

Wild parsnip is native to Eurasia and is thoroughly established as a weed in fields, waste places, and roadsides throughout the United States. It looks somewhat like wild carrot (Queen Anne's lace) but has yellow flowers.

Dittany, gas plant, fraxinella, or burning bush is a strong-smelling, showy, herbaceous perennial with pinnately divided leaves and large white, pink, or red flowers. It is native to Eurasia and is cultivated in northeastern United States as an ornamental shrub or hedge.

Phytophotodermatitis is frequently misdiagnosed as poison ivy or other contact dermatitis. The three prerequisites are moist skin from water or sweat, contact with the plant (direct or indirect), and then exposure to sunlight. Symptoms differ from contact dermatitis in that redness of skin and burning occur within 24 hours after exposure to plant and sun, and swelling and small to large blisters develop soon after. The intense residual redness persisting for months is diagnostic.

This type of dermatitis is not well known and may be more common than expected. Treatment of the symptoms would be the same as for contact dermatitis.

See Kingsbury (1964) for a discussion of photosensitization by plants.

INTERNAL POISONING

Plants considered as "internal poisons" are those that cause a chemical or physiological disturbance, or death, when eaten. True poisoning of this type, unlike allergies or dermatitis, does not depend on a previous sensitivity of the individual. The term "poisonous" as used here does not necessarily mean "fatal," but that which causes any symptoms of toxicity.

Much folklore surrounds the subject of plant poisoning, yet only a small percentage of all the plants known causes toxic reactions. A few are mildly toxic and a very few can be extremely so and even fatal if eaten in sufficient quantity. Some plants are harmful only if eaten in certain stages of their growth, or only certain parts of the plant may be toxic. Other plants may be poisonous in all stages of development, and all parts may be equally poisonous. Thus the particular type of plant, the stage of growth, the part eaten, the season of the year, the amount eaten, or the condition, age, and size of the person who eats it may all be important factors in determining the potential hazard. To judge from past cases, "berries," mushrooms, seeds, leaves, stems, flowers, and roots can all be real hazards to man—particularly to children.

Toxic chemicals are commonly classified as: alkaloids, polypeptides and amines, glycosides, oxalates, resins and resinoids, and phytotoxins. Many others are unique and are found in specific plants. For a discussion of these chemicals and their actions, see Kingsbury (1964).

First aid: What to do in case of internal poisoning

Call your physician immediately!

Be prepared to give him this information:
1. Name of plant if known.
2. How much and which parts of plant were eaten.
3. How long ago it was eaten.
4. Age of the individual.
5. Symptoms observed. All unusual symptoms should be carefully described.
6. A good description of the plant if the name is unknown. Save the specimen for later identification.

If a physician cannot be contacted

1. Have the individual drink a glass or two of water and then (if he is not unconscious or convulsive) try to produce vomiting by gagging the back of the throat with a finger or a blunt instrument (spoon, etc.), or by giving an emetic such as syrup of ipecac, warm salt water, mustard water, or soapy water.
2. Take the person to the nearest hospital emergency room or clinic. Be sure to take the plant along for identification if you have it.
3. The *Poison Control Center* in your area may be helpful if your physician is not available. These centers can provide information on proper therapy and may be able to aid in the identification of the plant. Locate the Poison Control Center for your area now. Telephone _____.

For identification of the plant

1. Use the index of this book if name is known or look at the illustrations.
2. Contact a botanist (plant taxonomist, if possible) at the nearest university, college, or high school; county agricultural agents, soil conservation agents (USDA), or museum curators may also be able to identify the plant.

Common poisonous plants

The plants included here are known, or strongly suspected, to have caused internal poisoning in humans. In addition, stock-poisoning plants could be harmful to children and adults if eaten in sufficient quantity. For a discussion of these see Kingsbury (1964) or a poisonous plant manual for your area, if available (see the Bibliography, pp. 148–153).

The fact that a plant is not mentioned in this book is no assurance that it is non-poisonous. Some uncommon ones have been omitted; others are yet to be recognized as dangerous.

The arrangement of the plants which follow is alphabetical by scientific name, within families arranged in a semievolutionary sequence from primitive to advanced. Any linear sequence such as this, however, is usually artificial in comparison to actual evolutionary relationships.

Common names of plants are unfortunately not standardized and can differ greatly among people within a region and between regions, which can lead to a great deal of confusion. Scientific names are standardized throughout the world and are given here for accuracy in linking the plant with the correct information on poisoning. A given plant species can have only one correct scientific name composed of two words followed by the name (or abbreviation) of the author who named it; for example, *Gloriosa superba* L. for the glory lily.

Occasionally scientific names are changed. For example, the well-known mistletoe of eastern United States has been known as *Phoradendron flavescens* for over a hundred years. Now we must change to *Phoradendron serotinum*. Why? Scientific name changes such as this are upsetting and discouraging to many people, yet the names of plants must conform rigidly with the International Code of Botanical Nomenclature and keep abreast of new and changing concepts in the science of botany. No name can be changed without a valid reason. In the case of mistletoe it was realized about ten years ago that *flavescens* was contrary to the Code and had to be changed to *serotinum*. In another case, poison oak and poison ivy are now considered sufficiently different from the sumacs (*Rhus*) to be called *Toxicodendron*. Therefore, rather than *Rhus radicans* for poison ivy we now find *Toxicodendron radicans*. Much printer's ink has been used denouncing "name changing" of well-known plants. Much less energy and adrenaline is expended learning the newer and more correct names than in resisting the changes.

The general habitat and distribution within continental United States and Canada is given for the native or naturalized plants. The presence of a plant in Alaska or Hawaii is noted separately. Cultivated plants have no specific distribution since many are now being grown outside their native climates in home greenhouses, on protected patios, or inside houses.

Notes on treatment are strictly intended for the physician alone, and any specific antidote should be administered only by a physician. Certain treatments, incorrectly given, could be as dangerous as the original poisoning. As will be noted, the treatment of plant poisoning is mainly symptomatic and supportive, and specific antidotes are neither available nor necessary except in rare cases.

ALGAE

Microscopic green plants known as algae are common inhabitants of surface water and are encountered in nearly all water exposed to sunlight for a period of time. While extensive growths of algae (blooms) may be a nuisance, most are not toxic. A few blue-green algae, however, may cause death to wild and domestic animals and illness or death to humans. Although poisoning of humans by algae seems fairly rare, some algae have been suspected as the possible cause of stomach and intestinal irritation among persons using a common water supply, or swimming in ponds with algal blooms. Water which is obviously polluted should be avoided.

Shellfish poisoning and the Redtide are caused by algae and have been serious problems on the Atlantic, Gulf, and Pacific coasts.

FUNGI

In addition to mushrooms, numerous other fungi may be dangerous. Some of these, such as ergot, are found growing commonly on various cereal grasses. See Kingsbury (1964) for a discussion of fungal toxicity and ergotism.

Poisonous mushrooms, or toadstools, are undoubtedly the most famous of all poisonous plants, yet they still cause numerous illnesses and deaths each year. Surprising as it may seem in a time when mushrooms can be bought at a reasonable price, vacuum-packed and sterile or neatly boxed and perfectly safe, in any gleaming supermarket, thousands of mycophagists still gather them in the woods and fields and on lawns. And equally surprising, despite all published warnings, a dismaying number of adults—the unwary and the knowledgeable—still pick and eat poisonous forms during the damp summer season.

The common name "toadstool" (*todesstuhl,* death's stool) is often given to mushrooms that are poisonous, but there is no recognizable difference between the poisonous toadstool and the non-poisonous mushroom. In fact there is no simple rule of thumb for making this distinction, and if anyone claims to have a tried and true method he is fooling himself. All such methods may work for a few species, but not for all. *Do not trust any of them,* for all so-called tests are myths and foolish nonsense. Remember you are gambling with life and death!

> There are old mushroom hunters
> And there are bold mushroom hunters,
> But there are no old, bold mushroom hunters.

There are several thousand species of mushrooms in the United States, but fortunately relatively few cause serious illness or death. There are three chief reasons for difficulties in distinguishing edible from poisonous forms. First, there are numerous species and the differences between them are rather subtle and require critical examination by the trained mycologist for correct identification. Second, many species are variable in their characteristics, and poisonous qualities may also vary depending upon the season, habitat, and geographical area. Third, poisonous and edible forms may not only look alike to the non-specialist but may grow together—even in the same fairy ring. In addition, the difficulties are magnified by variation in susceptibility among people.

No attempt will be made to describe the poisonous species, but a few of the more important and common types will be mentioned briefly. The common mushroom has a central stalk and cap at the top with flat plates (gills) on the lower surface of the cap (Figure 51). Rather than gills, some have minute pores in the lower surface of the cap. Puffballs differ by being more or less rounded without a stalk, and open at maturity by a hole at the top. The morels, another type of fleshy fungus, have a deeply ridged cylindrical top rather than a cap. There are poisonous species among all these types of fleshy fungi.

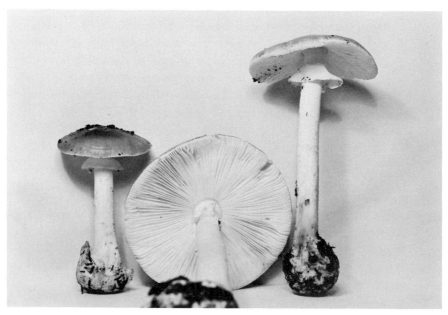

Figure 6. Destroying angel (*Amanita verna*) A deadly mushroom.   Courtesy of Dr. L. R. Hesler.

Amanita

The amanitas are found very commonly in fairy rings on lawns and in woods. They cause about 90 per cent of the deaths due to mushroom poisoning. There are numerous species in the United States and Canada, some quite edible, many poisonous. It is safest to avoid them all. In case of amanita poisoning, one or two bites may be fatal. Two species are shown in Figures 6 and 7.

Clitocybe

The jack-o'-lantern mushrooms (Figure 8) usually grow in large dense clusters at the base of trees or individually. Some are edible; some poisonous.

Lactarius

The milky-caps have a milky juice which exudes freely when the flesh is broken. This is a large group of common mushrooms found chiefly in woods. Some are edible, but all

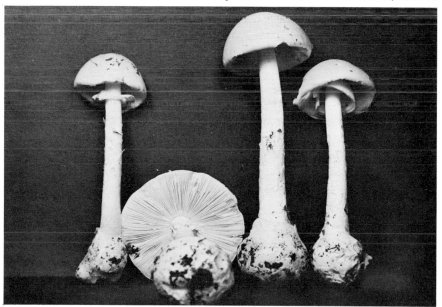

Figure 7. Browning amanita (*Amanita brunnescens*) Poisonous mushrooms. Courtesy of Dr. L. R. Hesler.

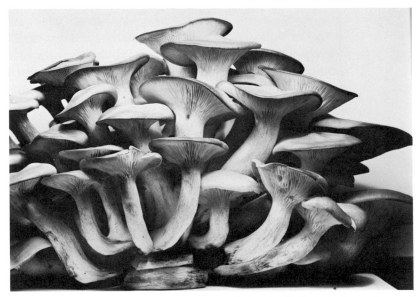

Figure 8. Jack-o'-lantern mushroom (*Clitocybe illudens*) A dense cluster of poisonous mushrooms. Photograph by Dr. L. R. Hesler, with permission of the University of Tennessee Press.

should be avoided. The milky juice, if tasted, may be mild at first, then quite acrid and peppery, lasting for some time.

Lepiota

The lepiotas are found very commonly in fairy rings on lawns and are very similar to amanitas. They are frequently large with the cap as much as 11 in. across. There are some edible species, but one of the very common types (Morgan's lepiota, Figure 9) causes many illnesses each year, and there are a few deaths on record. There is too much risk in trying to recognize the edible forms.

Russula

The russulas are quite common mushrooms which are white or often colored with red or purple caps. Some species are quite edible, some produce a very peppery taste, and a few are possibly poisonous.

Mushroom poisoning: The poisonous chemicals are either polypeptides in some or different alkaloids in others. The

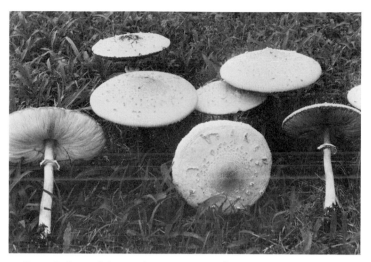

Figure 9. Morgan's lepiota (*Lepiota molybdites*) A common cause of mushroom poisoning. Photograph by Dr. L. R. Hesler, with permission of the University of Tennessee Press.

polypeptides are not destroyed by cooking. Symptoms may appear in either of two different forms. In one case there may be sudden stomach cramps, thirst, watering of eyes and mouth, sweating, difficult breathing, diarrhea, and vomiting. Mental disturbances, coma, and convulsions are also characteristic. In a second form there can be delayed symptoms (usually 6–24 hours) and a more deadly type of poisoning. This long asymptomatic period is often puzzling to the physician, and unless he is aware of this possibility an erroneous diagnosis and prognosis may be made. Vomiting and diarrhea are similar to the first type, and in addition liver damage and failure may result. Circulatory failure and coma usually follow within 2–10 days depending on the amount eaten.

The delicate and delicious taste of many mushrooms is not really worth the tremendous risk taken by eating wild forms.

To the physician: Gastric lavage (1:2000 tannic acid or 1:10,000 potassium permanganate solution) or an emetic; atropine; corticosteroids; peritoneal dialysis in serious intoxication; symptomatic and supportive.

FERNS

Eating of young fern "fiddleheads" or "crosiers" in salads or as a hot vegetable is fairly popular in some areas. Although some ferns are poisonous to livestock, none has been suspected of causing human poisoning. The picking of wild ferns should be restricted to those known to be edible in a particular region, and extreme caution should be taken not to confuse the young "fiddleheads" with young plants of the deadly poison hemlock or water hemlock.

CYCADS—*Cycadaceae*

Zamia spp. (Coontie, Florida arrowroot)

These are evergreen, fernlike, low plants with an underground stem and terminal female cones bearing orange-yellow naked seeds. They are found in dry sandy pinelands in Florida and are cultivated elsewhere in southern United States and Hawaii. Related cycads (*Macrozamia, Cycas, Dioon, Microcycas,* and others) are also cultivated as ornamentals in southern United States, Mexico, and Hawaii.

The fleshy seeds are poisonous if eaten in quantity. Paralysis and death have occurred from eating the seeds of *Cycas circinalis* (fern palm, false sago palm, crosier cycas). The seeds and roots are used for food in some areas but the alkaloid is washed out first.

To the physician: Gastric lavage or emesis; symptomatic.

YEW FAMILY—*Taxaceae*

Taxus spp.—Yew, ground hemlock

Description: Evergreen shrubs or small trees with narrow leaves which are alternate, stiff, ½–1½ in. long; seed single, green, ovoid, and nearly surrounded (except at the top) by a scarlet fleshy tissue (aril).

Occurrence: There are primarily two species (*T. cuspidata* Sieb. & Zucc. and *T. baccata* L.) cultivated as ornamental shrubs. The native species of eastern United States are *T. canadensis* Marsh. of rich woods from Canada southward in the mountains to North Carolina and Kentucky and *T.*

floridana Nutt. in rich woods of northwestern Florida. In western United States *T. brevifolia* Nutt. is found along mountain streams, gorges, and ravines below 7,000 ft. elevation from California to Alaska.

Poisoning: Most parts contain the poisonous alkaloid taxine, although the red aril around the seed is edible in small quantities. Symptoms from eating the leaves or seeds are diarrhea and vomiting, trembling, pupil dilation, difficult breathing, muscular weakness, and rapid collapse, coma, convulsions, and slow heartbeat; fatal if eaten in quantity.

To the physician: Gastric lavage or emesis; control pain with Demerol, otherwise symptomatic.

BANANA FAMILY—*Musaceae*

Strelitzia spp.—Bird-of-paradise

These small banana-like plants with showy birdlike flowers are occasionally cultivated in greenhouses, as house plants, or outside in Florida, Texas, California, and Hawaii. The leaves are straplike, and the colorful flowers (yellow and blue, white and purple, or blue and red) are clustered in a narrow boatlike leaf.

The 3-angled capsule and seeds are poisonous and cause vomiting, diarrhea, dizziness, and drowsiness if eaten.

To the physician: Gastric lavage or emesis; symptomatic.

LILY FAMILY—*Liliaceae*

Colchicum autumnale L.—Autumn crocus, meadow saffron, naked ladies

Description: Bulbous plants with long narrow basal leaves appearing in the spring; flowers white or light purple, in clusters appearing in the fall after the leaves have withered. This is not the commonly cultivated spring crocus.

Occurrence: Autumn crocus is cultivated in gardens and lawns throughout the United States and Canada and has become naturalized in some areas. It is a native of England, Europe, and Africa.

Poisoning: The alkaloid colchicine and related compounds

are found throughout the plant (leaves, flowers, seeds) although in highest concentration in the bulb. Children have been poisoned by eating the flowers. Eating of the bulb or flowers is followed by a burning pain in the mouth and kidney failure. Colchicine is used as a medicinal drug and also as an important tool in studies of plant genetics.

To the physician: Gastric lavage or emesis; shock therapy; symptomatic and supportive.

Convallaria majalis L.—Lily-of-the-valley

Description: Herbaceous perennial from a slender, running rootstock; leaves 2–3, basal, and to 1 ft. long; inflorescence a one-sided raceme of small, aromatic, nodding, white, bell-shaped flowers appearing in the early spring; fruit a red berry, but seldom forming.

Occurrence: This native of Eurasia is frequently cultivated in gardens or flower beds in the United States and Canada. It occasionally escapes near gardens. A related species (*C. montana* Raf.) is native in the rich woods of the high mountains of North Carolina, Tennessee, Virginia, and West Virginia.

Poisoning: Cardiac glycosides convallarin and convallamarin have a somewhat digitalis-like action causing an irregular heartbeat and stomach upset. Leaves, flowers, roots, and fruits are considered toxic.

To the physician: Gastric lavage or emesis; supportive; potassium, procainamide, quinidine sulfate, disodium salt of edetate (Na_2EDTA) have all been used effectively.

Gloriosa superba L.—Glory lily, climbing lily, gloriosa (Figure 10)

Description: Slender herbaceous plant or vine from a thick tuberous rootstock; leaves alternate or appearing opposite, simple, 4–7 in. long and ½–1 in. or more wide, with a terminal tendril-like tip; flowers on long stalks, 6-parted, each segment crinkled along the edges, yellow or red, turning upward, the 6 stamens and green pistil project downward; fruit an oblong capsule, 2–3 in. long.

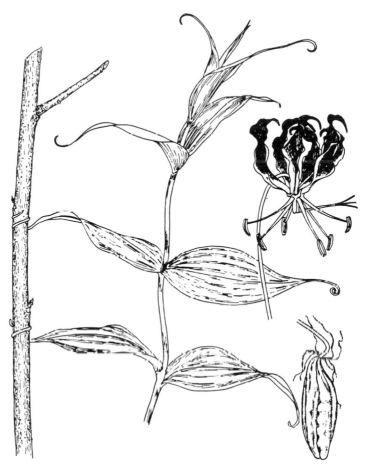

Figure 10. Glory lily (*Gloriosa superba*) A poisonous but attractive ornamental with upside-down flowers.   Courtesy of the Florida Agricultural Experiment Station.

Occurrence: Native of tropical Africa and Asia, the glory lily is frequently planted outside in Florida and Hawaii and is grown as a potted plant elsewhere in the United States.

Poisoning: All parts, particularly the tubers, contain alkaloids which are extremely poisonous, causing numbness of lips, tongue, and throat, diarrhea and vomiting, burning in the mouth and stomach, difficulty of breathing, convulsions, and death.

To the physician: Gastric lavage or emesis; shock therapy; symptomatic and supportive.

Hyacinthus orientalis L.—Hyacinth

The common garden hyacinth of lawn borders, flower gardens, and pots inside the house can be dangerous if eaten in quantity. The bulb is the most dangerous part, causing intense stomach cramps, vomiting, and diarrhea.

To the physician: Gastric lavage or emesis; symptomatic.

Ornithogalum umbellatum L.—Star-of-Bethlehem, snowdrop

Description: Herbaceous perennial from a bulb; leaves basal, linear with a light green midrib; stem leafless, to 1 ft. tall; flowers white and starlike, perianth parts 6, each with a green stripe on the back.

Occurrence: A native of Europe, this attractive plant is occasionally cultivated and has often escaped in waste places, roadsides, and lawns in the eastern and central United States, Canada, and Hawaii.

Poisoning: Various alkaloids are found in the bulb and aboveground parts and can cause nausea and intestinal disorders. Children have been poisoned by eating flowers and bulbs.

To the physician: Gastric lavage or emesis; symptomatic.

Veratrum viride Ait.—False hellebore, hellebore, Indian poke

Description: Herbaceous perennial, 3–8 ft. tall, from a thick vertical rootstock; leaves 3-ranked up the stem, 6–12 in. long and to 6 in. wide, oval, base sheathing the stem, with prominent veins and appearing pleated; flowers in a large terminal panicle with perianth parts 6, glandless, greenish-yellow, and hairy.

Occurrence: False hellebore is a native of rich woods or along streams and wet areas, from eastern Canada to Minnesota and south along the mountains into North Carolina, Georgia, and Tennessee. V. parviflorum Michx., recognized by its hairless flowers and narrower upper leaves, is also poisonous and is found in the mountains from West Virginia to Georgia. V. californicum Durand has whitish flowers and is found in moist meadows and slopes in the mountains of the Pacific coast and the Rockies south to New

Mexico. Additional species are found in Alaska and elsewhere.

Poisoning: Several alkaloids, such as veratrin, cause watering of the mouth, vomiting, diarrhea, stomach pains, general paralysis, and spasms. Severe cases may result in shallow breathing, slow pulse, lower temperature, convulsions, and death. An extract from the rootstock has been used for medicinal purposes, but known occurrence of human teratogens suggests that this is dangerous.

To the physician: Gastric lavage or emesis; activated charcoal; atropine, hypotensive drugs.

Zigadenus spp.—Black snakeroot, death camas

Description: Perennial herbs from a thick horizontal rootstock; stem to 3 ft. tall, smooth, leafy although most leaves are at the base; leaf blades narrow and grasslike, not stalked; flowers in terminal panicles, white or cream, the 6 perianth parts with 1–2 yellowish glands at the base on the upper side; fruit a 3-celled capsule.

Occurrence: Black snakeroot is frequent in open boggy or poorly drained areas. There are about fifteen species throughout the United States and Canada. It is assumed that all are more or less poisonous.

Poisoning: The alkaloids, such as zygadenine, are mainly concentrated in the bulb and cause muscular weakness, slow heartbeat, subnormal temperature, stomach upset with pain, vomiting, and diarrhea, and excessive watering of the mouth. Children have been poisoned by eating the bulbs and also the flowers.

To the physician: Gastric lavage or emesis; symptomatic, 2 mg. atropine subcutaneously and repeat as needed.

AMARYLLIS FAMILY—*Amaryllidaceae*

Narcissus spp.—Narcissus, jonquil, daffodil

This group of popular spring flowering plants so frequently found in yards and flowerpots may cause poisoning if eaten in quantity. The bulb is the most dangerous and will cause nausea, vomiting, diarrhea, trembling, convulsions, and may be fatal.

The related *Amaryllis (Hippeastrum)* and *Crinum,* both widely grown in warm areas for the attractive flowers, may also be dangerous.

To the physician: Gastric lavage or emesis; symptomatic.

ARUM FAMILY—*Araceae*

Dieffenbachia spp.—Dieffenbachia, dumbcane (Figure 11)

Description: Perennial herb with green stems 3–6 ft. tall; unstalked leaves large, oblong, green or often spotted, streaked, or mottled with white, lighter or darker green or yellow-green. There are many horticultural varieties with various color patterns of the leaf. The two species generally grown are *D. sequine* (Jacq.) Schott and *D. picta* (Lodd.) Schott.

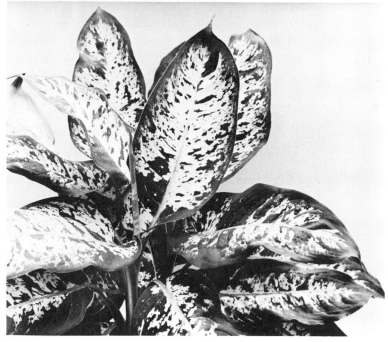

Figure 11. Dumbcane (*Dieffenbachia* sp.) An ornamental house plant with white-green variegated leaves.

Occurrence: These are tropical American plants widely cultivated as house plants, or planted outside in southern United States and Hawaii.

Poisoning: Severe burning in the throat and mouth is caused to some extent by numerous needle-like crystals (raphides) of calcium oxalate, but primarily by a protein (enzyme) or asparagine. In very severe cases swelling of the mouth and tongue may cause choking. Symptoms of nausea, vomiting and diarrhea may indicate the presence of additional toxins, but the details are unknown.

To the physician: Gastric lavage or emesis; symptomatic; give demulcents; cold packs to lips and mouth, antihistamines or epinephrine.

Other members of the arum family can be equally dangerous. The native and well-known Jack-in-the-pulpit, *Arisaema triphyllum* (L.) Schott, (Figure 12) found in rich woods throughout continental United States and southern

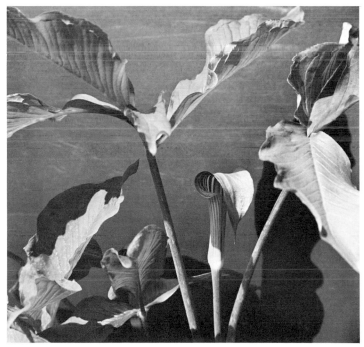

Figure 12. Jack-in-the-pulpit (*Arisaema triphyllum*) A well-known spring-flowering herb of rich woods with a dangerous root.

Canada, can cause similar injury to the mouth if the roots are eaten in quantity.

Philodendrons (*Philodendron* spp.) are among the most popular ornamental house plants (vines) introduced from the tropics. There are numerous horticultural forms with various leaf shapes, including the "cut-leaf" philodendron or monstera. The leaves and stems are dangerous if eaten in quantity.

Other genera such as *Alocasia, Colocasia* (elephant ears), *Caladium, Anthurium,* and others are found in the warm areas of the country, Hawaii, and Mexico.

PALM FAMILY—*Arecaceae, Palmae*

Areca catechu L.—Areca nut, betel nut

Description: A very tall (75 ft.) and slender palm with feather-like leaves to 3 ft. or more long; fruit oblong, to 2 in., orange or red, the outside soft and fleshy.

Occurrence; Betel nut palm is frequently planted as an ornamental in Florida, Hawaii, and the American tropics. The nut is chewed by South American and Asian natives for the narcotic effect.

Poisoning: The alkaloids arecolin, arecain, and others found in the seeds can cause pupil dilation, vomiting, diarrhea, convulsions, coma, and death.

To the physician: Gastric lavage or emesis; symptomatic, 2 mg. atropine subcutaneously and repeat as needed.

NUTMEG FAMILY—*Myristicaceae*

Myristica fragrans Houtt.—Nutmeg

This tall tree, planted widely in the tropics, is the source of the commonly used mace and nutmeg. In recent years nutmeg has become more popularly known as a narcotic— a mild hallucinogenic drug similar in action to marijuana (see p. 70).

Poisoning: Eating of nutmegs (the seeds) causes, in addition to some initial hallucinations and elation, stomach pain, redness of skin, dry mouth, drowsiness, stupor, double vision, and delirium. As few as two nutmegs can be fatal.

To the physician: 2–4 oz. mineral or castor oil, followed by gastric lavage and demulcents.

MOONSEED FAMILY—*Menispermaceae*

Menispermum canadense L.—Moonseed, yellow parilla (Figure 13)

Description: A perennial, woody, twining vine; stem smooth; leaves alternate and palmately lobed with 3–5 low rounded lobes, the stalk usually twisted; flowers greenish white in small axillary clusters; fruit a drupe, globular, black with a whitish wax on the surface, appearing in grapelike clusters, but each with a single seed which is grooved and crescent-shaped. The fruits are often confused with grapes. Grapes, however, have many seeds (rather than 1) and the leaves have 20 or more large pointed teeth on the margin (rather than 3–5 rounded lobes).

Figure 13. Moonseed (*Menispermum canadense*) Vine with poisonous grape-like berries.

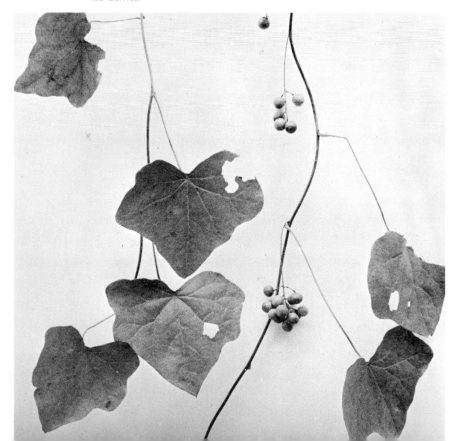

Occurrence: The moonseed vine is infrequent in moist woods and thickets from Canada south to Georgia and Oklahoma.

Poisoning: The fruits are dangerous if eaten in quantity. Birds eat these fruits readily, but contrary to popular belief what a bird eats is not necessarily safe for humans. Birds often feed without harm on fruits and seeds which are poisonous to other animals.

To the physician: Gastric lavage or emesis; symptomatic.

BUTTERCUP FAMILY—*Ranunculaceae*

Aconitum spp.—Aconite, monkshood, wolfsbane

Description: Perennial herb with ascending or nearly trailing stems; leaves alternate, palmately 3–9-lobed; flowers in terminal racemes or panicles, white to deep blue-purple, upper part hoodlike; fruit of 3–5 separate follicles.

Occurrence: *A. reclinatum* Gray (white flowers) and *A. uncinatum* L. (blue flowers) are native in rich woods, on slopes, and along creeks in the mountains and Piedmont of Georgia northward into Ohio and New York; *A. columbianum* Nutt. occurs in the high mountains and wet meadows in western Canada south to California and New Mexico. *A. nepellus* L. is European and commonly cultivated in gardens of the United States and Canada.

Poisoning: All parts of the plant contain the alkaloid aconitine and others. Symptoms are intense vomiting and diarrhea, muscular weakness and spasms, weak pulse, paralysis of the respiratory system, convulsions, and death in a few hours after eating the flowers, leaves, or roots.

To the physician: Gastric lavage or emesis; atropine, 2 mg. subcutaneously and repeat as needed; maintain blood pressure; artifical respiration.

Actaea spp.—Baneberry, white cohosh, snakeberry, doll's-eyes, coralberry (Figure 14)

Description: Perennial herb to 3 ft. tall from a thick rhizome; leaf blades large, spreading, pinnately divided, leaflets with toothed margins; flowers small and white, in a long-stalked terminal raceme; thick-stalked, white-berried *A. pachypoda* Ell. (*A. alba* of earlier authors), or thin-stalked, red- or white-berried *A. rubra* (Ait.) Willd.

Occurrence: Baneberry is native in rich woods and occurs from Canada south to Georgia, Alabama, Louisiana, Oklahoma, and the northern Rockies. The red-fruited western baneberry (*A. arguta* Nutt.) occurs from Alaska to central California, Arizona, Montana, and South Dakota.

Poisoning: All parts, but mostly the roots and berries, contain a poisonous glycoside or essential oil which causes acute stomach cramps, headache, increased pulse, vomiting,

Figure 14. Baneberry (*Actaea pachypoda*) Poisonous white fruit, or "doll's-eyes," on swollen reddish stalks.

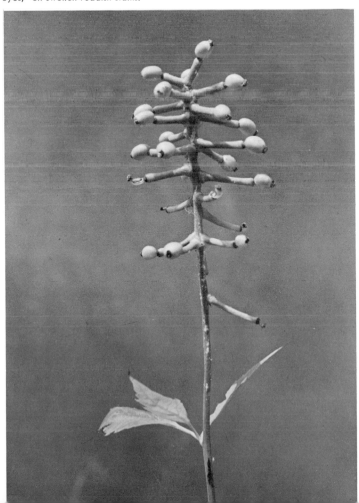

delirium, dizziness, and circulatory failure. As few as six berries can cause severe symptoms persisting for hours.

To the physician: Gastric lavage or emesis; symptomatic and supportive.

Delphinium spp.—Delphinium, larkspur, staggerweed

Description: Annual or perennial herbs 2–4 ft. tall; leaves finely palmately divided and on long stalks; flowers in a terminal raceme, white, pink, rose, blue, or purple; each flower with a spur projecting backward from the upper part; fruit a many-seeded follicle. The flowers may be double in some cultivated forms.

Occurrence: Larkspur is a native of rich or dry woods and rocky slopes throughout the country, but most common in western United States. These attractive plants are frequently cultivated in flower gardens.

Poisoning: The alkaloids delphinine, delphineidine, ajacine, and others are found mostly in the seeds and young plants. These alkaloids cause stomach upset, nervous conditions, depressions, and may be fatal if eaten in large quantities. Danger decreases as the plants become older.

To the physician: Gastric lavage or emesis; atropine, 2 mg. subcutaneously and repeat as needed; maintain blood pressure; artificial respiration.

Related plants which can cause similar poisoning are:

Adonis vernalis L.—Spring adonis, pheasant's eye
   Popular cultivated ornamental.
Anemone spp.—Anemone, windflower, pasqueflower, thimbleweed
   Native as well as cultivated.
Caltha palustris L.—Marsh marigold
   Native in Canada, northeastern, and north central United States.
Clematis spp.—Clematis, virgin's bower
   Native and cultivated throughout.
Helleborus niger L.—Christmas rose
   Cultivated ornamental.

Hydrastis canadensis L.—Golden seal
    Native in northeastern United States.
Ranunculus spp.—Buttercup, crowfoot
    Native throughout the area.

BARBERRY FAMILY—*Berberidaceae*

Podophyllum peltatum L.—Mayapple, mandrake
(Figure 15)

Description: Perennial herb with a creeping rhizome and thick fibrous roots; stem with 1 or 2 large, circular, 5–9-lobed leaves; flower solitary, nodding in the axil between the two leaves, with perianth white or cream; fruit a fleshy berry, turning yellow when ripe.

Occurrence: Mayapple is a well-known spring flower of the rich woods and open fields and pastures throughout southern Canada and the United States. It is often found in large clusters of many plants close together.

Poisoning: The resinoid podophyllin is found in the rootstock, stem, flower, leaves, and unripe fruit and can cause severe diarrhea with vomiting. Cases of poisoning are rare for the fruit can be eaten without harm when completely ripe

Figure 15. Mayapple (*Podophyllum peltatum*) A well-known herb with a dangerous unripe fruit. From *Flora of West Virginia*, courtesy of Dr. E. L. Core.

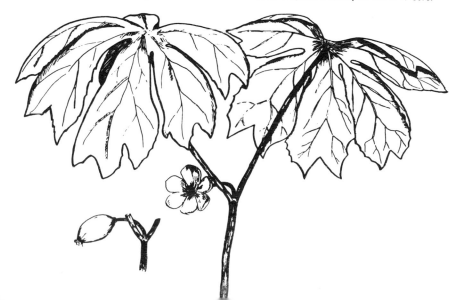

(yellow and soft) and if not eaten in quantity. Children have been poisoned by eating too much of the unripe fruit. An extract of the rootstock (podophyllin) is often used for medicinal purposes. Toxic effects on mitosis presumably could cause malformations in the human embryo, if taken by the mother during pregnancy.

To the physician: Gastric lavage or emesis; activated charcoal and antidiarrheal agents.

Caulophyllum thalictroides (L.) Michx.—Blue cohosh

Description: Perennial herb with a short knotty rootstock; stem simple, erect, bearing a large unstalked divided leaf and a raceme or panicle of small yellow-green or greenish purple flowers; the single ovary of each flower splits while young and exposes the 2 ovules, 1 of which develops into a dark blue naked seed.

Occurrence: This is a common plant of rich deciduous woods from Canada southward to Missouri and in the mountains and Piedmont to North Carolina and Alabama.

Poisoning: The leaves and seeds contain an alkaloid methylcytisine and also some glycosides which can cause severe stomach pains. Children have been poisoned by eating the bright blue seeds, although they are quite bitter to the taste. An extract from the rootstock is sometimes used for medicinal purposes.

To the physician: Gastric lavage or emesis; symptomatic.

POPPY FAMILY—*Papaveraceae*

Argemone mexicana L.—Mexican pricklepoppy, prickly poppy, thornapple

Description: An annual, whitish green herb with yellow juice; stem erect, usually branched, to 3 ft. tall; leaves alternate, thistle-like and prickly, the base of the leaf clasping the stem; flowers single and showy with 4–6 yellowish petals; fruit a prickly capsule opening near the top; seeds many and small.

Occurrence: Prickly poppy grows along fence rows and roadsides, in old fields and barnyards, and around buildings, in gardens and waste places. It is found from Florida to Arizona and northward into Pennsylvania and in Hawaii.

Poisoning: Various alkaloids (berberine, protopine, sanguinarine, and dihydrosanguinarine) are found in the leaves and seeds. *Argemone* has been a problem only when the seeds have contaminated home-ground corn, oats, or wheat. Symptoms are vomiting, diarrhea, difficulty of seeing, swelling throughout the body, fainting, and coma.

To the physician: Gastric lavage or emesis; symptomatic.

Chelidonium majus L.—Celandine, rock poppy

Biennial herb with reddish juice; flowers yellow. Celandine is a native of Eurasia and is established in moist soil from Canada to North Carolina and Missouri. Poisoning is the same as in *Argemone.*

Papaver somniferum L.—Common poppy, opium poppy

This erect annual with showy flowers and milky juice was once commonly planted in gardens and locally escaped in the United States. It is now unlawful to obtain, transport, or grow this species without a federal license. The common garden ornamentals are generally other species of *Papaver.*

Opium is a derivative of this species and comes from the juice of the young fruit. Poppy seeds used as topping of breads have only minute traces of the alkaloid and are not at all harmful. Eating the unripe fruit produces stupor, coma, shallow and slow breathing. The specific epithet *somniferum,* meaning "sleep bringing," indicates the long-known action of the extracts. Morphine and heroin, derivatives of opium, are the most vicious in their effects and claim an estimated sixty thousand addicts. Another derivative, commonly used to soothe colicky infants, is paregoric.

To the physician: Gastric lavage or emesis; strong coffee, support respiration, narcotic antagonists.

Sanguinaria canadensis L.—Bloodroot

Description: Flower white with many petals and conspicuous before the leaf unrolls; sap blood red.

Occurrence: Bloodroot is a very common and well-known

spring wildflower of rich woods from southern Canada to Florida and Texas.

Poisoning: The sanguinarine, present throughout the plant, causes vomiting, diarrhea, fainting, shock, and coma. This same chemical is extracted from the rootstock and used as a medicinal drug.

To the physician: Gastric lavage or emesis; symptomatic.

FUMITORY FAMILY—*Fumariaceae*

Dicentra spp.—Dicentra, bleeding heart, Dutchman's breeches, squirrel corn, turkey corn (Figure 16)

Description: Glabrous perennial, short-stemmed herbs from a cluster of small tubers or a stout fleshy rootstock; leaves pinnately divided, the ultimate segments deeply lobed and very narrow; flowers white or pink, in a raceme or panicle; corolla 2-spurred or saclike on the upper side; fruit a capsule.

Occurrence: There are a number of species native to rich woods in various parts of the United States and Canada; others are cultivated as garden or potted ornamentals.

Poisoning: The alkaloids protopine and others, found throughout the plant, cause trembling, staggering, convulsions, and labored breathing. Large quantities can be fatal.

To the physician: Gastric lavage or emesis; symptomatic.

POKEWEED FAMILY—*Phytolaccaceae*

Phytolacca americana L.—Pokeweed, pokeberry, poke, ink-berry, pigeonberry (Figure 17)

Description: Large shrublike herb to 8 ft. tall, stem green to red or purple; leaves alternate, oblong, to 1 ft. long, decreasing in size toward the top of the plant, margin not toothed; flowers in a drooping or erect raceme, white; fruit a round, purple-black juicy berry, about ½ in. across, drooping, or erect in *P. rigida* Small.

Occurrence: A native weed throughout eastern United States and southern Canada. It is common in open fields, along fences, roadsides, in waste places, and disturbed areas

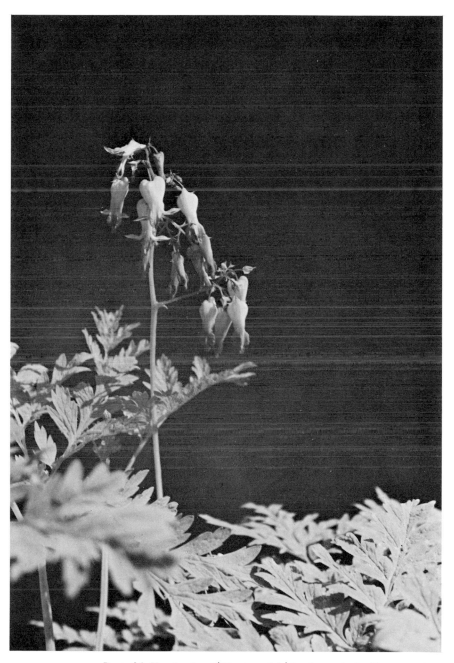

Figure 16. Bleeding heart (*Dicentra eximia*) A poisonous herb of flower gardens.

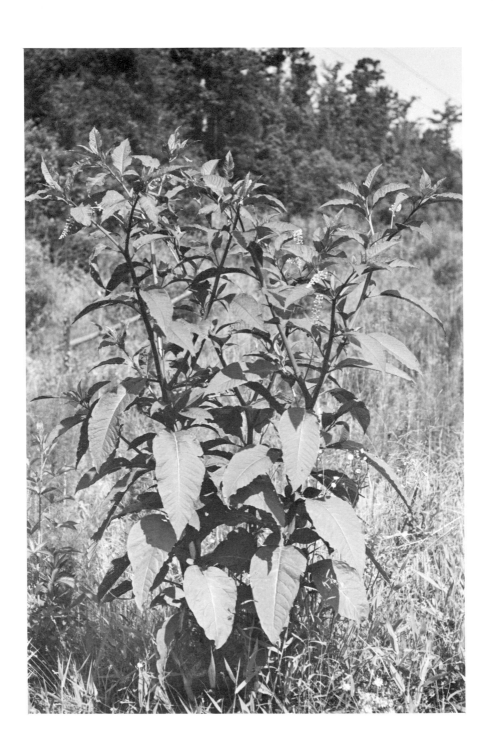

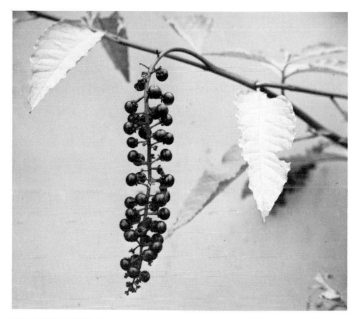

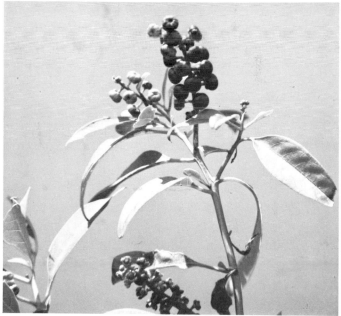

Figure 17. Pokeweed (*Phytolacca americana*) A common large weed of disturbed areas; stalks of berries show difference between *P. americana* (top) and *P. rigida* (bottom).

in general. It is also an occasional weed on the West Coast and in Hawaii. *P. rigida* is found along the coastal dunes and marshes from North Carolina to Texas and inland in Florida. Three additional species are found in Hawaii.

Poisoning: The poisonous principle is in highest concentration in the rootstock, less in leaves and stems, and least in the fruits. Eating of the poisonous parts causes severe stomach cramps and pain, nausea with persistent vomiting, diarrhea, slowed and difficult breathing, weakness, spasms, severe convulsions, and death.

Young tender leaves and stems of poke are frequently eaten as cooked greens. If thoroughly cooked (in two waters) the leaves are quite edible. Nevertheless, this is one of the most dangerous poisonous plants in the United States, because people eat the leaves without proper and complete boiling, or accidentally pull up the roots with the leaves. A few (1–10) berries are generally harmless to adults and older children, although more than 10 can cause serious poisoning. Infants, however, can be seriously or fatally poisoned by eating a very few berries. Cooked berries are edible and used for pies without harm.

The roots and sometimes fruits are used as a source of a drug for medicinal purposes, but its usefulness is highly questioned.

To the physician: Gastric lavage or emesis; symptomatic and supportive. Peripheral plasmacytosis with potential immunosuppressive properties has been reported recently.

PINK FAMILY—*Caryophyllaceae*

Agrostemma githago L.—Cockle, corn cockle (Figure 18)

Description: Annual erect weed to 3 ft. tall with white silky hairs; leaves opposite, 2–4 in. long, narrow; flowers single, about 1 in. across, 5-parted with pink or purplish petals; fruit a capsule with many black seeds each with a pitted surface.

Occurrence: Corn cockle is native of Europe and is widely established in the United States and southern Canada as a weed in cultivated grain fields and waste places. It is

sometimes cultivated as an ornamental annual. Because of
the difficulty of screening the seeds from wheat, it is
particularly common in wheat fields and from these has
invaded roadsides and other disturbed areas. Highly contaminated wheat which cannot be sold causes annual losses
of millions of dollars to wheat growers.

Poisoning: The seeds contain githagenin which causes
severe stomach pain with vomiting and diarrhea, dizziness,

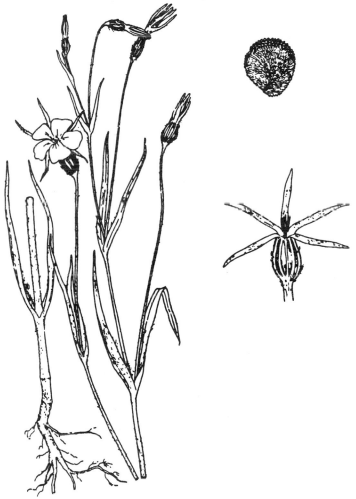

Figure 18. Corn cockle (*Agrostemma githago*) A frequent weed of grain fields
with poisonous seeds.   Courtesy of the Missouri Agricultural Experiment Station.

weakness, and slow breathing. The seeds are of particular danger as a contaminant of home-ground corn, wheat, or oats.

To the physician: Gastric lavage or emesis; symptomatic and supportive.

FOUR-O'CLOCK FAMILY—*Nyctaginaceae*

Mirabilis jalapa L.—Four-o'clock, marvel-of-Peru

Description: An herb with erect, much-branched stems from 1–3 ft. tall; leaves opposite, deep green, stalked, ovate, 2–6 in. long, pointed at the tip; flowers about 1 in. across, opening late in the afternoon or in very cloudy weather, white to red, yellow or striped, the 1–2 in. tubular portion 5-lobed at the top, and a 5-lobed calyx-like leaf at the base; fruit a leathery, 5-ribbed achene.

Occurrence: A native of tropical America and Mexico, four-o'clocks are cultivated in the United States as a favorite ornamental. They have escaped cultivation in parts of southern United States, California, and lower elevations of Hawaii.

Poisoning: The roots and seeds are the cause of acute stomach pain, vomiting, and diarrhea in children.

To the physician: Gastric lavage or emesis; symptomatic.

CACTUS FAMILY—*Cactaceae*

Lophophora williamsii (Lemaire) Coult.—Peyote, mescal, mescal buttons (Figure 19)

Description: A small (1–3 in. across) hemispherical, spineless, fleshy cactus from a large, branched perennial rootstock, and with low rounded sections each bearing a tuft of yellow-white hairs at the summit; flower from the center of the plant, small and white to rose-pink; fruit a pink berry when ripe; seeds black. The taste is very bitter and disagreeable.

Occurrence; A native of southern Texas and northern Mexico, it is shipped into other parts of the country as a narcotic. Peyote is recognized officially as a narcotic by some states, which makes it unlawful to possess any amount

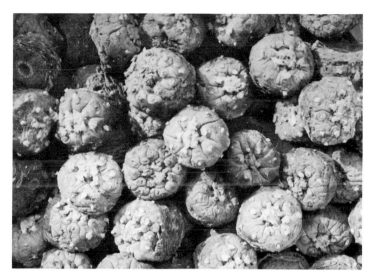

Figure 19. Peyote (*Lophophora williamsii*) A collection of "buttons." Courtesy of the North Carolina State Bureau of Investigation.

of the plant. Many states, however, have no legal restrictions at this time.

Poisoning: Peyote has long been used by Indians and other groups in their religious rites. The Aztecs considered it sacred, and it is still a sacramental feature of the Native American Church which claims two hundred and fifty thousand adherents among Indians of the western states.

Chewing fresh or dried pieces of the "buttons" (individual aboveground plants) produces illusions and hallucinations with extraordinary colored visions, but also headache, pupil dilation and blurred vision, muscular relaxation and dizziness, circulatory depression, loss of sense of time, wakefulness, and often severe stomach pain with vomiting and diarrhea. Several alkaloids (mescaline, lophophorine, etc.) are known, their action being somewhat similar to, although less potent than, the recently publicized LSD (lysergic acid diethylamide). It has been shown that peyote causes chromosome damage, as does LSD, making them extremely dangerous during pregnancy.

Unfortunately it has become popular for many, particularly

high school or college students and the "hippie" society, to experiment with various hallucinogenic or psychedelic drugs —peyote, marijuana, LSD, etc. Although peyote may not cause a physiological addiction, the psychotic reactions and long-range effects are dangerous, and it can be psychologically habit forming. Peyote should be considered a dangerous poisonous plant and a narcotic in the legal sense.

To the physician: Early gastric lavage or emesis if thorough vomiting does not occur naturally.

BUCKWHEAT FAMILY—*Polygonaceae*

Rheum rhaponticum L.—Rhubarb

Rhubarb, commonly known for the edible leaf *stalks* (petioles), is quite poisonous if the leaf *blades* are eaten. Stomach pains, nausea, vomiting, weakness, difficulty of breathing, burning of mouth and throat, internal bleeding, coma, and death can occur. The poisonous substance is possibly a soluble oxalate with an additional unknown toxin.

Rhubarb is frequently grown in flower or vegetable gardens in northern United States and Canada and southward in the mountains to Georgia, Alabama, Colorado, and in Hawaii.

To the physician: Gastric lavage or emesis with lime water, chalk, or calcium salts; calcium gluconate; parenterally force fluids; supportive.

BOXWOOD FAMILY—*Buxaceae*

Buxus sempervirens L.—Boxwood, box

Description: Evergreen shrub with angular or winged stems; leaves simple, opposite, oval, ½–¾ in. long, leathery and dark green above and pale below with a whitish midrib.

Occurrence: Boxwood is cultivated extensively as a hedge or shrub in this country. There are many horticultural varieties as well as additional species in cultivation from the Old World.

Poisoning: The leaves and twigs contain buxene, which causes stomach pains, vomiting, and diarrhea. Large amounts may cause convulsions and death.

To the physician: Gastric lavage or emesis; symptomatic.

SAXIFRAGE FAMILY—*Saxifragaceae*

Hydrangea spp.—Hydrangea

Description: Shrubs to 10 ft. tall; leaves opposite and simple, elliptical, stalked, lobed or not, margins coarsely toothed; flowers in dense, rounded to flat-topped clusters to 1 ft. across; each flower white, pink, or blue, 4–5-lobed; sterile flowers, with an expanded calyx which is very showy and to 1 in. across, occurring at the periphery or throughout the cluster.

H. arborescens L.—Hydrangea, mountain hydrangea, sevenbark

These are native shrubs of dry or moist woods or rocky woods and hillsides, New York to Iowa, south to Florida and Arkansas. The flowers are white. There are a number of of native and cultivated varieties of this species.

H. macrophylla Ser.—Hydrangea

This native of Japan, with many horticultural varieties, is commonly cultivated as an ornamental shrub for the large pinkish or blue flowers, or white, and in rounded clusters.

H. quercifolia Bartr.—Oak leaf hydrangea, sevenbark

This species is native in mixed forests of Florida, Alabama, Mississippi, Tennessee, and Georgia and is occasionally cultivated outside this native area. The flowers are white and the leaves are deeply lobed.

H. radiata Walt.—Snowy hydrangea, silverleaf

This is quite similar to *H. arborescens* (and often included with it) except for the back of the leaf, which is very white and hairy. It is limited to the southern Appalachians.

Poisoning: The leaves and buds contain hydrangin, a cyanogenic glycoside, which under certain conditions causes nausea, vomiting, and diarrhea. The roots are sometimes used as a source of a medicinal drug.

To the physician: Gastric lavage or emesis; treat for cyanide poisoning.

ROSE FAMILY—*Rosaceae*

Prunus serotina Ehrh.—Black cherry, wild cherry (Figure 20)

Description: Tree 15–60 ft. tall; bark of twig very bitter to taste; leaves alternate, simple, 1–5 in. long, deciduous, the margin finely toothed; leaf stalk with 2 glands at the upper end just beneath the blade; blade hairless and shiny above and hairless below except for hairs along lower part of midrib; flowers small, white, 5-parted with many stamens, in racemes; fruit a dark purple or black drupe.

Occurrence: Black cherry is a very common tree in woods and fields, along fence rows, and in waste places throughout eastern North America.

Poisoning: All parts, particularly bark, leaves, and seeds, contain the cyanogenic glycoside amygdalin which yields hydrocyanic (prussic) acid upon hydrolysis brought on by partial wilting. The fruit is edible if the seeds are discarded. Poisoning can lead to difficult breathing, paralysis of the voice, twitching, spasms, coma of short duration, and death. Cyanide poisoning can occur suddenly and without many obvious symptoms. Children have been poisoned by eating the seeds, chewing on twigs, and making "tea" out of the leaves. The bark and sometimes the dried fruit are used as a source of a medicinal drug.

Related species of *Prunus* may also be poisonous: cherry, cherry laurel or laurel cherry, plum, almond, peach—native and cultivated forms. Seeds of the common apple or crab apple (*Malus* spp.) are similarly poisonous.

To the physician: Gastric lavage or emesis; treat for cyanide poisoning.

Rhodotypos tetrapetala Makino—Jetbead, jetberry bush

This is a commonly cultivated shrub in the northern part of the United States. The shining black drupes, in clusters of 4 with 4 spreading jagged sepals below, persist into the winter and are quite attractive. The drupes contain amygdalin, as *Prunus* above.

To the physician: Gastric lavage or emesis; treat for cyanide poisoning.

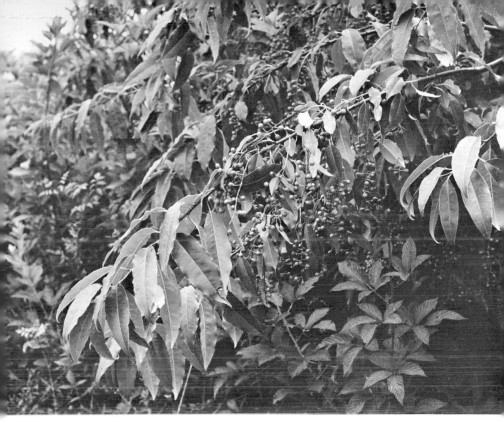

Figure 20. Black cherry (*Prunus serotina*) A common tree of eastern United States; small photograph below shows characteristic bark of the trunk.

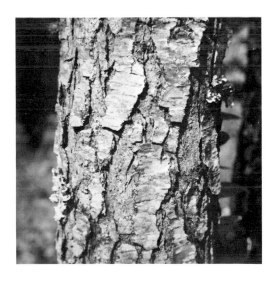

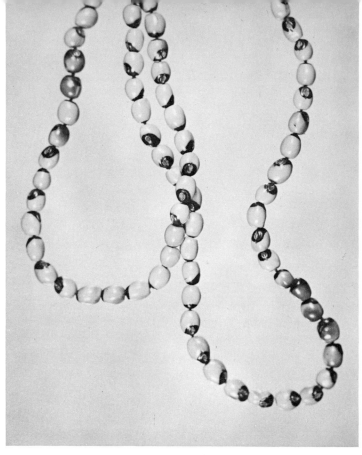

Figure 21. Jequirity pea or rosary pea (*Abrus precatorius*) A portion of a necklace made of the beautiful but deadly red and black seeds.

PEA FAMILY—*Fabaceae, Leguminosae*

Various beans and peas are among our most important vegetables and cover crops. Within the same family we find some of the most dangerous of the poisonous plants.

Abrus precatorius L.—Jequirity pea, precatory bean, rosary pea, crabseye, prayer bean, love bean, lucky bean (Figure 21)

Description: A vine of tropical areas; leaves alternate and divided with small leaflets; flowers red to purple or white; fruit a legume to 1½ in. long, with ovoid seeds about ¼ to ⅜ in. long, glossy, bright scarlet over three-fourths and jet black over one-fourth of the area.

Occurrence: This deadly vine is occasionally found growing in central and southern Florida and the Keys in citrus groves and waste places as a weed. The seeds are so colorful and attractive that they are frequently used in rosaries, necklaces, leis, and various toys. They are sold in stores or brought back into the United States by those traveling in Central America, Mexico, the West Indies, or Hawaii. They are favorite playthings of children and therefore of extreme danger.

Poisoning: The seeds contain abrin, a phytotoxin, which causes severe stomach pain in 1–3 days, with nausea, vomiting, severe diarrhea, weakness, cold sweat, drowsiness, colic, weak and fast pulse, coma, circulatory collapse, and trembling. The seeds are harmless if not chewed because of their impermeable seed coat which prevents absorption of the chemical into the body. If the seed is thoroughly chewed, however, one seed is said to be fatal to a child. The poison can also be taken in through a pricked finger while stringing the beans.

To the physician: Gastric lavage or emesis; maintain circulation and correct for hemolytic anemia with blood transfusions; keep urine alkaline and treat for uremia; saline cathartics and control dehydration.

Daubentonia punicea (Cav.) DC.—Rattlebox, purple sesbane, false poinciana

Description: Deciduous shrub or small tree to 12 ft. tall; leaves alternate, 4–8 in. long, pinnately divided with 12–40 leaflets, each with a minute pointed tip and untoothed margin; flowers orange to red in drooping, axillary clusters near the ends of the branches; legume about 3 in. long, 4-winged, with a cross-partition between the seeds and not splitting open.

Occurrence: Native of Mexico and planted as an ornamental shrub, rattlebox has often escaped in various disturbed habitats in the southeastern United States Coastal Plain.

Related plants with poisonous seeds are *Sesbania* (sesban) and *Glottidium* (bladderpod, bagpod), found mostly in the southeastern United States along roadsides and in fields.

Some sesbans are found in Hawaii and from California to Central America.

Poisoning: The seeds contain saponins which cause depression, diarrhea, and rapid pulse which may not develop until 24–48 hours after eating. In severe cases weakness, difficult breathing, and death can occur. The flowers also are poisonous if eaten.

To the physician: Gastric lavage or emesis; symptomatic.

Dolichos lablab L.—Hyacinth bean, lablab

Description: A twining vine with alternate, divided leaves each composed of 3 broad ovate leaflets, 3–6 in. long and sometimes equally broad, and rather abruptly pointed at the tip; flowers white, pinkish, or purple, in clusters of 2–4 along a raceme, each flower ½–1 in. long; legume flat, 2–5 in. long with 3–5 black or white seeds.

Occurrence: This vine is native of the Old World tropics but now is widely cultivated for food in South America and elsewhere in the tropics. Hyacinth bean has been introduced into North America as an attractive ornamental vine and has become naturalized in some areas, particularly in Hawaii.

Poisoning: The pods and seeds are cooked thoroughly (2–4 waters) for food in the tropics. Insufficient boiling causes poisoning from a cyanogenic glycoside.

To the physician: Immediate gastric lavage or emesis; treat for cyanide poisoning.

Gymnocladus dioica (L.) K. Koch—Kentucky coffee tree

Description: Large, rough-barked tree to 80 ft. tall; leaves alternate, to 3 ft. long, twice pinnately divided with leaflets ovate and margins untoothed; fruit a flat legume 3–6 in. long with 4–7 flat broad seeds and sticky pulp between them.

Occurrence: This handsome tree is native in moist woods from Canada to Alabama and Oklahoma and is occasionally cultivated elsewhere in the United States as a lawn or street tree.

Poisoning: The legume, with the pulp between the seeds, can be confused with the more common honey locust

(*Gleditsia triacanthos*), which also has pulp between the seeds but is not poisonous. The legume of the honey locust is much longer (8–15 in.) and often twisted or curved and has sweet pulp and a thinner wall; honey locust is also typically thorny although there is a thornless variety. The seeds and pulp of the Kentucky coffee tree contain the alkaloid cytisine which causes stomach and intestinal disorders with diarrhea, vomiting, irregular pulse, and coma. The seeds have been used in the past as a substitute for coffee.

To the physician: Gastric lavage or emesis; activated charcoal, artificial respiration, and oxygen.

Laburnum anagyroides Medic.—Golden chain

Description: Shrub or small tree; leaves alternate, trifoliate, long-petioled; flowers golden yellow, in long drooping racemes; fruit a long flat legume.

Occurrence: The beautiful golden chain tree is native in southern Europe and is cultivated as an ornamental flowering shrub or tree, mainly in northern United States and southern Canada.

Poisoning: The flowers and seeds contain cytisine, which causes excitement, stomach and intestinal irritation with nausea, severe vomiting, and diarrhea, irregular pulse, convulsions, coma, and death if large quantities are eaten.

To the physician: Gastric lavage or emesis; symptomatic; activated charcoal, artificial respiration and oxygen.

Lathyrus spp.—Sweet pea, everlasting pea, vetchlings, singletary pea

Sweet peas are vines commonly cultivated for the showy flowers in erect racemes. They often escape cultivation in many areas. The seeds are poisonous and can cause paralysis, slow and weak pulse, shallow breathing, and convulsions. See Kingsbury (1964) for a review of lathyrism.

The wild sweet pea (*Hedysarum mackenzii* Rich.) of Alaska and Canada is reported as poisonous.

To the physician: Gastric lavage or emesis; symptomatic.

Poinciana gilliesii Hook.—Poinciana, bird-of-paradise

This showy, non-spiny shrub is occasionally cultivated as a large potted plant, or outside in extreme southern United States and Hawaii. The leaves are alternate, with numerous very small leaflets; flowers light yellow with long red stamens, in a terminal raceme; fruit a legume to ¾ in. wide and 4 in. long. The green seed pods cause serious stomach and intestinal irritation if eaten.

To the physician: Gastric lavage or emesis; symptomatic.

Pongamia pinnata Wight—Pongam

This tree or woody climber from India is cultivated occasionally in southern Florida, southern California, and Hawaii. The leaves are pinnately divided with 5–7 pointed and stalked leaflets and hang from drooping branches; flowers lavender or pinkish, fragrant, and hang in clusters like wisteria; the short pointed woody pod generally contains a single seed.

The seeds and roots are considered poisonous and are used in parts of India to poison fish.

To the physician: Gastric lavage or emesis; symptomatic.

Robinia pseudoacacia L.—Black locust (Figure 22)

Description: A large tree with alternate, odd-pinnately divided leaves; leaflets 7–25, each oval or elliptical and with a smooth margin; 2 spines present at the base of the leaf stalk; flowers white, in drooping racemes; fruit a flat legume.

Occurrence: Black locust is a common tree in dry woods and along roadsides and fence rows in southern Canada, eastern and central United States. It is also naturalized in the Pacific states from Washington to central California.

Poisoning: Inner bark, young leaves, and seeds contain robin, a phytotoxin, and robitin, a glycoside, which cause dullness and depression, vomiting, diarrhea, weak pulse, and coldness of arms and legs. Children have been poisoned by sucking on fresh twigs, eating inner bark, and eating seeds.

To the physician: Gastric lavage or emesis; symptomatic and supportive, keep urine alkaline.

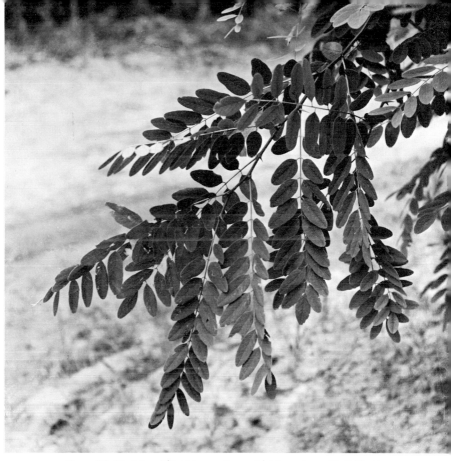

Figure 22. Black locust (*Robinia pseudo-acacia*) A large tree with divided leaves and drooping clusters of white flowers; below, twin stipular spines at base of the leaf.

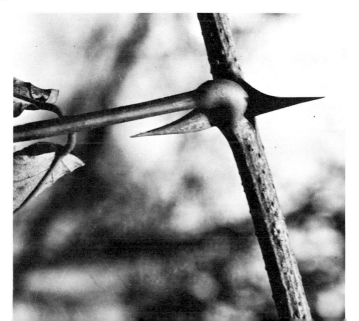

Sophora secundiflora (Ort.) Lag.—Mescal bean

> Description: Evergreen shrub or tree to 40 ft. tall; leaves stalked, alternate, 4–6 in. long, pinnately divided with 7–9 leaflets, shiny yellow-green above and silky below when young; pealike flowers violet-blue, very fragrant, and about 1 in. long, in 1–sided racemes; legume woody and white-hairy, the seeds ½ in. long and bright red.
>
> Occurrence: The mescal bean is found on ranges, hills, and in canyons from southwestern Texas and New Mexico into Mexico, and is grown widely in southern United States for its graceful foliage and attractive flowers.
>
> Poisoning: The seeds contain poisonous alkaloids which cause vomiting, diarrhea, excitement, delirium, and coma. One seed, thoroughly chewed, is sufficient to cause death in a child. These have long been used as a medicine and narcotic by Indians in Mexico and the southwest.
>
> To the physician: Gastric lavage or emesis; symptomatic.

Vicia faba L.—Fava bean, broad bean, horse bean, English bean, Windsor bean

> Description: An annual vine; leaves alternate, divided with 2–6 leaflets, each 2–4 in. long, without tendrils; flowers dull white with purplish blotch in center, one to several in the leaf axils; fruit a long legume, to 12–14 in., thick and angled and with many seeds; the seeds flattened and angled or nearly globular, brown to green, purplish, or black.
>
> Occurrence: This plant is widely and commonly cultivated as an ornamental vine in various areas of southern United States. The fava bean is a native of Europe and is often grown for food in some areas. The beans are appearing on the United States markets both canned and frozen.
>
> Poisoning: The beans (seeds) raw or cooked can cause severe hemolytic anemia appearing 2–3 days after eating. This condition, known as "favism," produces a profound anemia, headache, dizziness, diarrhea, nausea and vomiting, abdominal pain, fever, and death in some cases. Inhalation of pollen from the flowers can cause headache and dizziness

in 2–3 hours. Favism is found only in certain individuals of the Negro race (about 10 per cent) and in about 1 per cent of white Caucasians of Greek or Italian origin. This inherited trait has been known for centuries and is characterized by a deficiency of an enzyme known as G-6-PD (glucose-6-phosphate dehydrogenase). It is most serious in children and most common in boys. The beans may be eaten without danger by those not carrying this genetic trait.

To the physician: Gastric lavage or emesis; blood transfusion if necessary; keep urine alkaline.

Wisteria spp.—Wisteria (Figure 23)

The wisteria vine, or shrub or small tree in some cultivated forms, is commonly cultivated and is often escaped mainly in the southeastern United States. The pealike flowers are white to purple in large, showy, drooping racemes. The seeds and pods have been found to cause stomach and intestinal disturbances with repeated vomiting, stomach

Figure 23. Wisteria (*Wisteria sinensis*) A beautiful and popular vine of the southeastern United States; on the right, pod with poisonous seeds,

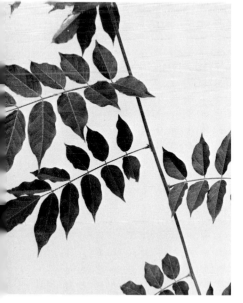 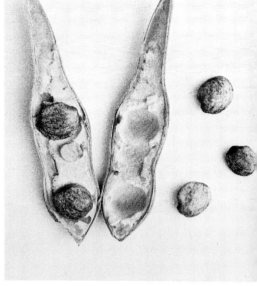

pain, diarrhea, and collapse. Two seeds are sufficient to cause serious illness in a child.

To the physician: Gastric lavage or emesis; symptomatic.

MULBERRY FAMILY—Moraceae

Morus rubra L.—Red mulberry

Description: Deciduous trees with alternate, simple, toothed, palmately veined leaves, unlobed, mitten-shaped, or 3-lobed; flowers small, in cylindrical short racemes, the sexes separate; fruit a juicy short-cylindric cluster of small drupes, resembling a blackberry, turning from white to red to purple-black as it ripens.

Occurrence: Mulberry is a native tree of rich woods, along fence rows, and in waste places from Vermont to Michigan and south to Florida and Texas. The related *M. alba* L. (white mulberry) is a native of Asia and is cultivated and escaped throughout the area.

Poisoning: The *unripe* fruits and milky sap in leaves and stems cause hallucinations and stimulation to the nervous system with stomach upset.

To the physician: Gastric lavage or emesis; symptomatic.

HEMP FAMILY—*Cannabaceae*

Cannabis sativa L.—Marijuana, marihuana, hemp, hashish, pot (Figure 24)

Description: A coarse, rough-stemmed annual 6–12 ft. tall; leaves long-stalked, palmately divided into 3–7 leaflets which are narrow and coarsely toothed; leaves opposite below and alternate in the upper portion of the stem; flowers small and green, crowded on axillary branches.

Occurrence: A native of central and western Asia, marijuana is occasionally planted illegally in the United States, Hawaii, and Canada as a narcotic. It is also infrequently found in waste places and roadsides as a persistent weed in Canada southward to Georgia and Colorado.

Poisoning: The narcotic and toxic resins are found throughout the green or dried plants, although the parts are most dangerous during hot summer weather. The effects caused by drinking the extract, chewing the plant parts, or smoking "reefers" or the extracted resins have been known for more than two thousand years. Symptoms are exhilaration, hallucinations, delusions, blurred vision, poor co-ordination, stupor, and coma.

In comparison to other hallucinogenic drugs, marijuana is fairly mild and may be classed with the heavenly blue and pearly gates morning glory seeds or nutmeg. More potent is the mescaline from peyote (see pp. 56–57) and psilocybin and bufotenine from certain mushrooms. The most potent is the chemical LSD (lysergic acid diethylamide), the basic ingredient for which is lysergic acid from ergot, a cereal fungus. Nevertheless, marijuana is one of the most commonly used drugs both in Canada and in the United States. The real danger in marijuana is that persons who start using this narcotic often turn to stronger habit-forming drugs.

Federal and state laws prohibit the possession of living or dried parts of marijuana, both in the United States and in Canada.

To the physician: Gastric lavage or emesis; symptomatic and supportive.

Figure 24. Marijuana
(*Cannabis sativa*) An
illegally planted narcotic.
From *Flora of West Virginia*,
courtesy of Dr. E. L. Core.

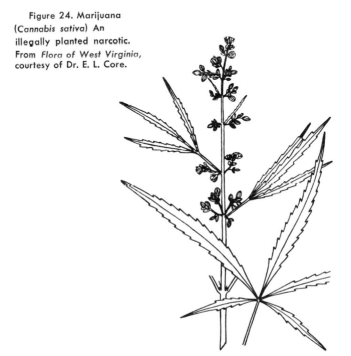

OAK FAMILY—*Fagaceae*

Fagus spp.—Beech

Beechnuts have caused poisoning in Europe, and although the American beech (*Fagus grandifolia* Ehrh.) is reported as edible, the nuts should not be eaten in quantity, particularly by children. Beech is one of the characteristic trees of the eastern deciduous forest and common in rich woods and ravines, or cultivated as an ornamental. The European beech, *F. sylvatica* L., is occasionally cultivated in northern United States as an ornamental.

Quercus spp.—Oak

Acorns and young shoots cause severe poisoning in livestock in certain areas. Although not reported as causing poisoning in humans, raw acorns may be dangerous if eaten in quantity. There are some sixty species in the United States and Canada, forming the most common trees of many forest associations.

MEZEREUM FAMILY—*Thymelaeaceae*

Daphne mezereum L.—Daphne, spurge laurel

Description: Deciduous shrub 1–4 ft. tall; leaves simple, alternate, 2–3 in. long, hairless; flowers in clusters of 2–5 along branches of the previous year and appearing before the leaves, lilac-purple, fragrant, silky outside, ½ in. or less long; fruit a round drupe ¼ in. across, leathery and scarlet. Variety *alba* has white flowers and yellow drupes.

Occurrence: Daphne is cultivated as an ornamental shrub throughout the United States and has escaped in the Northeast and in eastern Canada. Other species are widely cultivated as ornamentals.

Poisoning: All parts, but primarily the very attractive drupes, contain a glycoside in which the aglycone is dihydroxycoumarin which causes burning or ulceration of the throat and stomach, vomiting, internal bleeding with bloody diarrhea, weakness, coma, and death. Only a few drupes can be fatal to a child.

To the physician: Demulcents, gastric lavage or emesis; symptomatic and supportive.

LECYTHIS FAMILY—*Lecythidaceae*

This family of tropical trees is known mainly for the ornamental or edible nuts. Some are infrequently cultivated in southern Florida and Hawaii as ornamentals for their curious fruits (cannonball tree, monkey pots). Others are best known in North America through the importation of the edible and delicious Brazil nuts.

The nuts of some of the ornamental forms are said to cause nausea and chills if eaten in quantity.

MYRTLE FAMILY—*Myrtaceae*

Rhodomyrtus tomentosa (Ait.) Hassk.—Hill gooseberry, downy myrtle

The downy myrtle is a small, hairy shrub to 5 ft. tall, a native of Asia, grown to a limited extent in southern California, Texas, and Florida. In Hawaii it is considered a noxious weed. The fruit is a rounded berry, dull pink with numerous small flat seeds embedded in soft pulp of rather sweet flavor. The fruits are occasionally eaten raw or made into pies or jam. It is not poisonous, but the danger lies in the possible incorrect identification of the related species below.

R. macrocarpa Benth. of Australia, called finger cherry or Queensland loquat, is poisonous. The fruits contain high quantities of saponin, causing temporary or permanent blindness if eaten. The danger from the finger cherry was considered so serious in 1915 that the Department of Education in Queensland, Australia, issued illustrations and descriptions of the plant to be displayed in all schools. In 1945 there were twenty-seven cases of permanent blindness reported among soldiers in New Guinea. This particular species is not cultivated in North America, to our knowledge.

HOLLY FAMILY—*Aquifoliaceae*
Ilex spp.—Holly

There are a number of native and cultivated, deciduous and evergreen, holly shrubs and trees. Although they are not generally considered very poisonous, the red or black berries do cause disturbances such as vomiting, diarrhea, and stupor when eaten in quantity. They should be considered dangerous to small children.

One of the native species along the southeastern United States coast is called *I. vomitoria,* which indicates the potential action of the extract, long known and used (although questionably) as "black drinks" by the Indians. Early settlers in the Southeast enjoyed a harmless and very mild brew from the leaves called "yaupon tea."

To the physician: Gastric lavage or emesis; symptomatic.

STAFF-TREE FAMILY—*Celastraceae*

Euonymus spp.—Burning bush, strawberry bush, hearts-a-bustin', spindle tree, wahoo

Description: Shrubs or woody climbers with opposite, simple leaves; flowers small and greenish maroon; fruit conspicuous after splitting, with the seeds and capsule wall of contrasting shades of red, orange, or yellow.

Occurrence: There are a number of species of native shrubs of damp woods throughout the United States. Other species from Europe and Asia are cultivated extensively as ornamental shrubs or woody climbers. The related climbing bittersweet, *Celastrus scandens* L., is a vine or climbing shrub found in woods and thickets of damp soil from Ontario to Manitoba and south to North Carolina and New Mexico; it is also cultivated as an ornamental. The seeds may be poisonous to children if eaten in quantity.

Poisoning: The leaves, bark, and attractive seeds contain a poisonous principle which can cause vomiting, diarrhea, weakness, chills, coma, and convulsions. No cases have been reported from North America, but poisoning is known in Europe and all species should be suspected of potential danger.

To the physician: Gastric lavage or emesis; symptomatic.

BUCKTHORN FAMILY—*Rhamnaceae*

Karwinskia humboldtiana Zucc.—Coyotillo

> Description: Woody shrub or small tree with opposite, stalked leaves, 1–3 in. long with distinct straight lateral veins; flowers small, greenish, in lateral clusters; fruit a rounded drupe, turning brownish black when ripe, and about ½ in. across.

> Occurrence: This shrub is found on dry hills, in canyons, or in river valleys from southwestern Texas into Mexico and southern California.

> Poisoning. The fruit and seeds have long been known by the Indians to cause paralysis a few days after eating. Children have been poisoned by eating these colorful fleshy fruits.

> To the physician: Gastric lavage or emesis; symptomatic.

Rhamnus spp.—Buckthorn

> Buckthorns are opposite-leafed shrubs which contain glycosides which are fairly strong laxatives. One species has the name *R. cathartica,* which indicates the potential action of the extract. Another, *R. purshiana,* is the source of cascara—a commonly used laxative.

> Poisoning, by eating the black, juicy, berry-like fruit and the leaves, has been reported from Europe.

GRAPE FAMILY—*Vitaceae*

Parthenocissus quinquefolia (L.) Planch.—Virginia creeper (Figure 25)

> Description: A vine with alternate, long-stalked leaves which are palmately divided into 5 leaflets, each toothed on the margin, elliptical, and pointed; fruit a small blue berry, several in a cluster.

> Occurrence: Virginia creeper is a well-known and very common vine of woods, fields and disturbed areas throughout the eastern United States and westward to Wyoming, Colorado, and Arizona (including the western *P. vitacea* Hitchc.).

> Poisoning: This common plant is highly suspected of

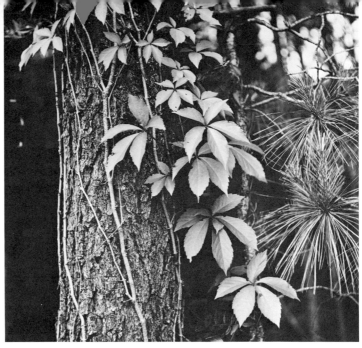

Figure 25. Virginia creeper (*Parthenocissus quinquefolia*) A common vine growing here on the trunk of a pine tree. Note *five* leaflets per leaf as compared with *three* in poison ivy. The berries are dangerous.

causing poisoning and death of children from eating the berries. The details are not known.

To the physician: Gastric lavage or emesis; symptomatic.

MISTLETOE FAMILY—*Loranthaceae* or *Viscaceae*

Phoradendron serotinum (Raf.) M. C. Johnston [*P flavescens* (Pursh) Nutt.].—Mistletoe (Figure 26)

Description: Semiparasitic evergreen shrub with greenish branches; leaves opposite, simple, oblong, ½–1½ in. long, leathery; fruit a small white berry.

Occurrence: Mistletoe is a common parasite on the branches of various types of trees from New Jersey and southern Indiana southward to Florida and Texas. Additional species are found in western United States and southward. Mistletoe is the state flower of Oklahoma.

Poisoning: Gerarde's *Herball* (London, 1597) states that mistletoe "inwardly taken is mortall, and bringeth most greevous accidents, the toong is inflamed and swolne, the mind is distraughted, the strength of the hart and wits faile." The berries contain toxic amines which cause acute stomach

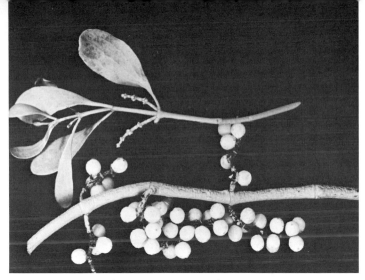

Figure 26. Mistletoe (*Phoradendron serotinum*) A frequent parasite in trees; the white berries used for Christmas decorations are poisonous. USDA Photograph.

and intestinal irritation with diarrhea and slow pulse. Since mistletoe is a favorite plant for Christmas decorations, care should be taken that the berries are kept out of reach of small children.

To the physician: Gastric lavage or emesis; supportive; potassium, procainamide, quinidine sulfate, disodium salt of edetate (Na$_2$EDTA) have all been used effectively.

MAHOGANY FAMILY—*Meliaceae*

Melia azedarach L.—Chinaberry, China tree, Chinaball tree (Figure 27)

Description: Deciduous tree 20–40 ft. tall; leaves alternate, 1–3 ft. long, twice pinnately divided with leaflets 1–2 in. long and toothed on the margins; flowers in large terminal panicles, lilac-colored and small; fruit a drupe, ½ in. across, cream or yellowish and persisting throughout the winter.

Occurrence: A native of Asia, Chinaberry is frequently cultivated as an ornamental and has escaped freely and become naturalized in old fields and pastures, around farm buildings and homes, along borders of woods and fence rows. It is quite common in the southern United States and at lower altitudes in Hawaii.

Poisoning: The fruits, as well as "tea" made from the

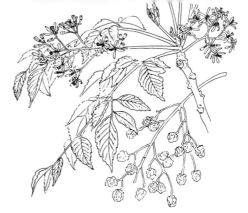

Figure 27. Chinaberry (*Melia azedarach*) A tree with large divided leaves, small lilac flowers, and yellowish wrinkled berries. Courtesy of the Florida Agricultural Experiment Station.

leaves, are poisonous to children if eaten in quantity. The toxic principle is probably a resinoid which causes narcotic effects, vomiting and diarrhea, paralysis, irregular breathing, and very marked symptoms of suffocation. Six to 8 fruits caused death in a young child.

To the physician: Gastric lavage or emesis; symptomatic.

SOAPBERRY FAMILY—*Sapindaceae*

Blighia sapida Koenig—Akee

This stiff-branched tree with pinnately divided leaves is native in western Africa. It was named for Captain W. Bligh, commander of the "Bounty." Akee is grown in the tropics, including southern Florida, for its edible fruit, which is a capsule with thick hard walls, roundish or triangular in outline, about 3 in. across, and straw-colored to red. Each of the 3 cells of the capsule contains 1 round shining black seed with a white oily base (aril). The white aril of the mature fruit is prepared and eaten without harm.

Poisoning: Acute vomiting followed by convulsions, coma, and death occurs when one eats the fruit wall, the black seeds, the white aril of unripe fruit, or the rancid spoiled aril.

To the physician: Gastric lavage or emesis; symptomatic and supportive; intravenous administration of glucose is important because of severe hypoglycemia produced by peptides.

BUCKEYE FAMILY—*Hippocastanaceae*

Aesculus spp.—Buckeye, horsechestnut

Description: Trees and shrubs; leaves deciduous, opposite, palmately divided with 5–9 leaflets on a long stalk; leaflets widest at the middle or above and toothed on the margins; flowers yellow, red, or white, 4–5-parted, in terminal panicles appearing with the leaves; fruit a 3-valved capsule with a thick leathery husk enclosing 1–6 brown shiny seeds with a large pale scar.

A. californica (Spach) Nutt.—California buckeye

Flowers white, stamens longer than the 5 equal petals; fruit rough. This is a shrub or small tree of dry hillsides and canyons in the Pacific Coast Range and the Sierras. The related *A. parryi* Gray is found in northern Baja California, Mexico.

A. glabra Willd.—Ohio buckeye

Flowers yellow, stamens longer than the 4 petals; fruit spiny. This tree is found in woods and along streams in western Pennsylvania to southern Michigan and Nebraska south to Arkansas and Texas.

A. hippocastanum L.—Horsechestnut

Flowers white, in broad panicles; fruit spiny. This very beautiful tree is cultivated in the United States and Canada. There are a number of horticultural forms and hybrids. It is a native of southeastern Europe, and a favorite ornamental in Europe and England.

A. octandra Marsh.—Yellow buckeye

Flowers yellow with flower stalks glandular hairy, stamens shorter than the petals; fruit smooth. Yellow buckeye is a large tree of the Ohio River valley and in the Appalachians southward to northern Alabama and Georgia. It is one of the characteristic trees of rich woods of the southern Appalachians.

A. parviflora Walt.—Bottlebrush buckeye

Flowers white, stamens very long, inflorescence a long

narrow panicle; fruit smooth. This is an uncommon shrub native in the Coastal Plain of southern Georgia and Alabama, but it has been cultivated occasionally northward.

A. pavia L.—Red buckeye, firecracker plant

Flowers typically red, except for a yellow form in Texas; fruit smooth. This beautiful shrub is found in low woods of the Coastal Plain from North Carolina to Florida and west to Texas.

A. sylvatica Bartr.—Painted buckeye (Figure 28)

Flowers yellow, the flower stalks not glandular; fruit smooth. Painted buckeye is a shrub of moist woods in the Piedmont from southern Virginia to Alabama and southeastern Tennessee.

Poisoning: The leaves, flowers, young sprouts, and entire seeds contain the glycoside esculin. Children have been poisoned by eating the seeds, or making "tea" from the leaves and twigs. Symptoms are nervous twitching of muscles, weakness, lack of co-ordination, dilated pupils, vomiting, diarrhea, depression, paralysis, and stupor. Amounts as little as 1 per cent of the child's weight may be poisonous. Roots, branches, and fruits have been used to stupify fish in ponds. Honey, mainly from the California buckeye, is also poisonous.

To the physician: Gastric lavage or emesis; symptomatic.

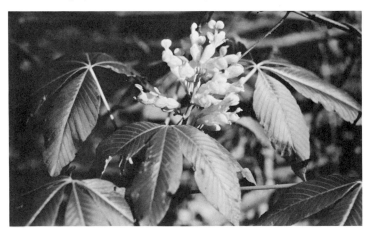

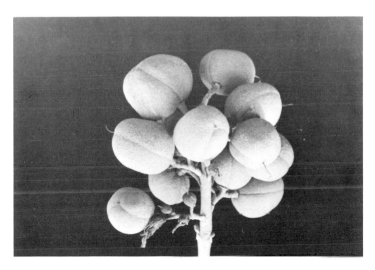

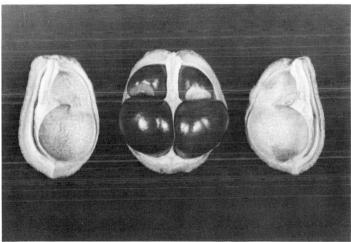

Figure 28. Painted buckeye (*Aesculus sylvatica*) Shrub with five leaflets, yellow flowers, and poisonous brown seeds in leathery husks.

Erythroxylon coca Lam.—Coca

Coca is an evergreen shrub or tree with alternate, simple leaves, small flowers which vary from yellow to white, and red to brownish drupes. It is a native in South America and is extensively cultivated in South America, Ceylon, India, and Java. Coca is occasionally cultivated in southern Florida,

California, and Hawaii and could be of danger if the leaves are eaten in quantity by children.

Coca has a long and fascinating history, known back to pre-Incan graves of the sixth century. It was known as the "divine plant" of the Incas during the tenth century in Peru. Chewing of coca leaves increases energy, decreases hunger, and dulls pain and generally enables the user to work harder and with less food than he could otherwise. The Spanish, who conquered Peru in the early sixteenth century, took advantage of these properties and encouraged coca chewing among the Indians so that they could endure the slavelike work in the silver and gold mines.

Today coca claims more addicts than any other narcotic—fifteen million in South America, mostly in Peru. The coca addict chews the leaves two to three times a day, particularly before work, along with lime or alkaline ashes of certain plants which aid in the extraction of the narcotic alkaloids. This drug has, through many generations, been of primary importance in the psychological disturbances and general racial degeneration in the Andean region and is of major social and political concern today in those regions.

In addition to numerous aromatic and sweet alkaloids, coca leaves contain cocaine, used extensively as a local anesthetic since the late nineteenth century. Now, synthetic substitutes have generally replaced its use by the physician. Cocaine, however, is a potent and dangerous habit-forming alkaloid. The "dope fiend" of the novelist is a cocaine addict.

Coca leaves are also important in the soft-drink industry. In 1887, A. G. Candler of Atlanta, Georgia, obtained a formula from Brazil for medical purposes, and the drink, made from a combination of coca leaves and the cola nut (a plant of the chocolate family), was obtainable by prescription only from his wholesale drug business. As the stimulating properties of the coca-cola drink became known, it gradually developed into the prosperous business of today. The coca-cola syrup contains caffeine from the cola nut plus the fatty acids from the coca leaves after the alkaloids have been removed. The drink is therefore quite lacking in the narcotic effects received from chewing the coca leaves.

Poisoning: Cocaine produces various symptoms depending on the individual. Some people are affected by very small amounts with headache, rapid respiration, delirium, coma, or convulsions with wide dilation of pupils. Persons addicted to cocaine eventually develop digestive disturbances, muscular twitching, insomnia, mental, moral, and physical deterioration, often resulting in death.

To the physician: Gastric lavage or emesis; symptomatic, activated charcoal.

CALTROP FAMILY—*Zygophyllaceae*

Guaiacum officinale L.—Lignum vitae

This small evergreen tree of the American tropics yields the valuable lignum vitae, an extremely hard and heavy wood, and also the resin guaiacum used for medicines, stains, and as a chemical indicator. The resin in the wood and fruit is poisonous if eaten in quantity. The tree is occasionally planted in southern Florida, Mexico, southern California, and Hawaii as an ornamental.

GINSENG FAMILY—*Araliaceae*

Hedera helix L.—English ivy, ivy

Description: Woody, climbing, or creeping vine with numerous short aerial roots; leaves evergreen, leathery, alternate, and simple, stalked, the blade palmately veined and variously shaped in different horticultural varieties; flowers small and greenish; fruit a small, 3–5-seeded black berry in clusters 4–10.

Occurrence: A native of Europe, ivy is very frequently planted as an ornamental vine. It occasionally escapes or persists in various habitats throughout most of the United States, Hawaii, and southern Canada.

Poisoning: The leaves and berries contain the saponic glycoside hederagenin. Symptoms are excitement, difficult breathing, and coma. The related *Aralia spinosa* L., Hercules' club or devil's walkingstick, of the eastern United States has black berries that may also be poisonous if eaten in quantity.

To the physician: Gastric lavage or emesis; symptomatic and supportive, paraldehyde (2–10 cc.) IM, oxygen and artificial respiration as necessary.

CARROT FAMILY—*Apiaceae, Umbelliferae*

Cicuta maculata L.—Water hemlock, spotted water hemlock, spotted cowbane (Figure 29)

Description: Perennial herbs 3–7 ft. tall with clustered, short and thickened tuberous roots and hairless, purple-striped or -mottled stems which are hollow except for

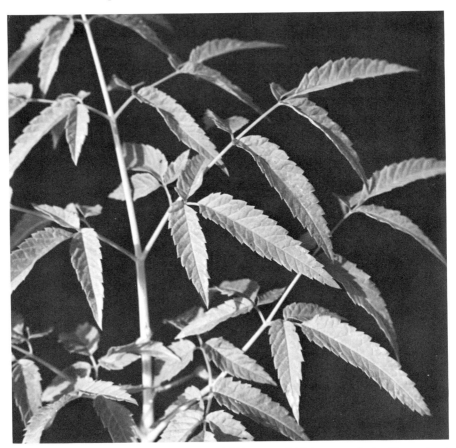

Figure 29. Water hemlock (*Cicuta maculata*) A common herb with very large divided leaves, flat-topped clusters of small white flowers, and a cluster of tuber-like roots; note cavities at base of the stem.   Drawing of root a USDA Photograph.

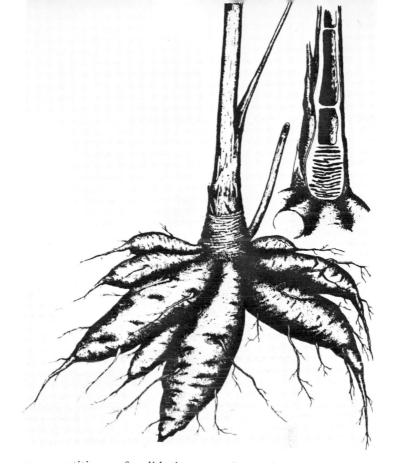

cross-partitions of solid tissue at the nodes; the rootstock exhibits several chambers or thin cavities separated by cross-partitions, as seen in a lengthwise cut through the root at the base of the stem; leaves alternate, leaf stalks clasping the stem, blade 2–3 pinnately divided, to 2 ft. long; leaflets narrow, 1–4 in. long, the margins toothed and the major veins ending in the notches between the teeth rather than in the tips of the teeth; flowers small, white, in terminal flat-topped or umbrella-shaped clusters (umbels); fruits small, dry, and ribbed.

Occurrence: Water hemlock is found in moist habitats in thickets, meadows, along stream banks, around spring heads, in marshes, seepage areas, and roadside ditches throughout eastern United States and Canada. Other species of *Cicuta* occur in various areas over the entire United States, Alaska, and Hawaii.

Poisoning: The poisonous chemicals are found mostly in the rootstock and much less in the aboveground parts of the plant. The root is extremely poisonous, and one mouthful of root is sufficient to kill a grown man. It is so often mistaken for wild parsnip or wild artichoke that deaths are frequent. Children have been poisoned by making peashooters and whistles from the hollow stems. Symptoms are diarrhea, violent convulsions and spasms, tremors, extreme stomach pain, dilated pupils, frothing at mouth, delirium, and death.

To the physician: Gastric lavage or emesis; symptomatic; control convulsions with parenteral short-acting barbiturates.

Conium maculatum L.—Poison hemlock, poison fool's parsley (Figure 30)

Description: A biennial herb with a hairless purple-spotted or -lined hollow stem to 8 ft. tall by the second

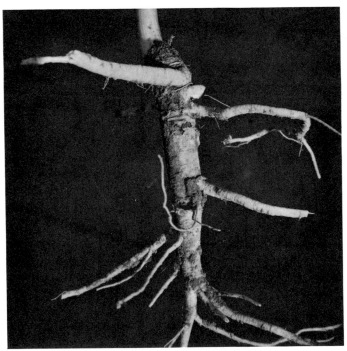

Figure 30. Poison hemlock (*Conium maculatum*) A European herb of historical fame and a weed in the U.S. The leaves are very deeply divided into minute leaflets (USDA Photograph). The root is a single taproot. (See facing page.)

season; taproot long, solid, and turnip-like; leaves large, 3–4 times pinnately divided, alternate and with a clasping stalk; the leaflets very minute; flowers and fruit similar to those in *Cicuta*.

Occurrence: A native of Eurasia, poison hemlock is found occasionally as a weed in waste places, marshy areas, and

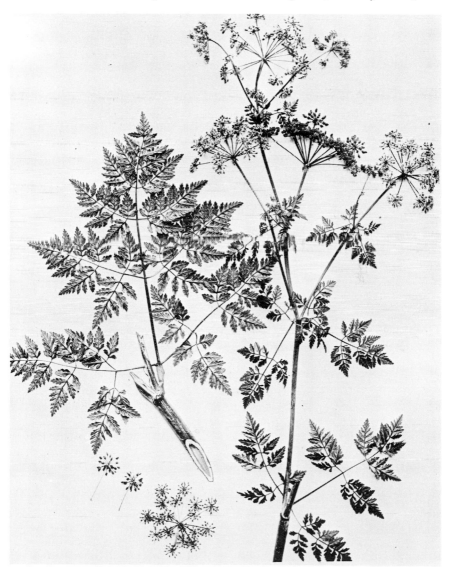

roadside ditches throughout eastern United States, the Rocky Mountains, Pacific coast, and southern Canada.

Poisoning: This is one of the most noted of the poisonous plants since it was used by the early Greeks as a regal means of dying. The offenders would crown themselves with a garland of flowers; then, with a brave smile and appropriate final remarks to those gathered, they would gulp the cup of hemlock. So went Socrates and others. It is not such a regal death in the United States, where, quite by accident or ignorance, the leaves are sometimes mistaken for parsley or the seeds are mistaken for anise. The taste is quite unpleasant, however, and toxic quantities are seldom consumed. Symptoms are vomiting and diarrhea, muscular weakness, nervousness, trembling, dilation of pupils, weak pulse, convulsions, coma, and death. The poisonous principles are coniine and other alkaloids; they occur in greatest concentration in the seeds and root.

To the physician: Gastric lavage or emesis; saline cathartic; keep airway clear, oxygen and artificial respiration; anticonvulsive therapy.

Note: The two hemlocks just mentioned (*Cicuta* and *Conium*) should not be confused with the trees called hemlock, which are conifers of the genus *Tsuga* and not at all poisonous.

MUSTARD FAMILY—*Brassicaceae, Cruciferae*

Various members of the mustard family, both wild and cultivated throughout the area, can cause vomiting and diarrhea if eaten raw and in quantity by small children. The roots are the most dangerous. Cabbage, mustard, kale, brussels sprouts, cauliflower, broccoli, rutabaga, turnip, radish, cress, horseradish, and stock are examples.

GOURD FAMILY—*Cucurbitaceae*

Momordica charantia L.—Wild balsam apple, balsam pear, bitter gourd

Description: Climbing or creeping vine; leaves alternate, deeply palmately lobed, to 2½ in. across; flowers yellow, tubular, small; fruit warty, orange-yellow, 1½–5 in. long, oblong, and tapered at both ends, the seeds and pulp red.

Occurrence: This little vine is found on the Coastal Plain from Florida to Texas in sandy soils and waste grounds. It is cultivated in gardens in Hawaii.

Poisoning: The seeds and wall of the fruit contain a purgative causing vomiting and diarrhea. One fruit is sufficient to cause severe stomach and intestinal disorders in a child. The red fleshy covering around the seed (aril) is harmless and is sucked from the seeds by children and adults alike.

To the physician: Gastric lavage or emesis; symptomatic.

SPURGE FAMILY—*Euphorbiaceae*

Aleurites fordii Hemsl.—Tung oil tree, tung nut (Figure 31)

Description: Deciduous tree to 25 ft. tall; leaves alternate, simple, long-stalked, heart-shaped, to 10 in. long, margins

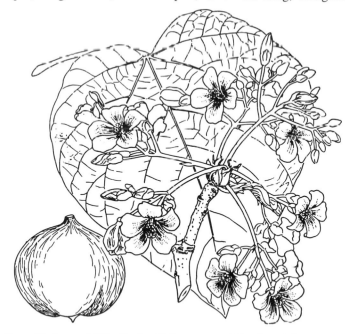

Figure 31. Tung nut (*Aleurites fordii*) Tree commercially planted for tung oil. The attractive seeds are extremely dangerous. Courtesy of the Florida Agricultural Experiment Station.

smooth; flowers pale pink to white, petals 5–7, in large panicles; fruits on drooping stalks, 2–3 in. across, globular, turning brown at maturity, seeds 3–7 with rough seed coats.

Occurrence: Tung oil tree is a native of China and is planted in the Gulf Coast region from northern Florida to Texas. Large commercial orchards are planted for the tung oil. Trees are also planted in the same area as ornamentals and for shade. Related species are less toxic. The candlenut (*A. moluccana* Willd.) has edible seeds which are roasted and eaten in Hawaii, but raw seeds are poisonous.

Poisoning: All parts of the tung oil tree contain a saponin and phytotoxin. Symptoms from eating the attractive seeds are very severe stomach pain with vomiting, diarrhea, weakness, slowed breathing, and poor reflexes. Death may occur. A single seed can cause severe poisoning, and cases are frequent where the trees are common.

To the physician: Gastric lavage or emesis; symptomatic; control convulsions with parenteral short-acting barbiturates.

Euphorbia spp.—Spurge

Description: Numerous species of upright or prostrate herbs or shrubs, sometimes cactus-like; juice milky and acrid; leaves alternate or opposite, simple, smooth or toothed; "flowers" (cup-shaped structures bearing minute male and female flowers inside) greenish and often bearing glands or white petal-like appendages on the rim of the cup; fruit a globose, 3-lobed capsule on a long stalk extending from the cup.

E. corollata L.—Flowering spurge

Slender, diffusely branched herb; leaves 1–2 in. long, green, and smooth margined; white petal-like appendages of the "flower" conspicuous. This is a common native weed of fields, woods, and disturbed areas throughout eastern United States.

E. cyparissias L.—Cypress spurge

Glabrous perennial with erect stems to 1 ft. tall; leaves crowded above, narrowly linear, ½–1 in. long. A native of Eurasia, this popular border plant is cultivated in gardens or yards and occasionally escapes in various parts of the United States.

E. lathyris L.—Caper spurge, mole plant, sassy jack

Glabrous annual to 3 ft. tall; leaves mainly opposite, 1½–5 in. long; capsule about ½ in. across. This is a native of Europe which is occasionally cultivated and sometimes escapes as a weed in various areas throughout the United States.

E. marginata Pursh—Snow-on-the-mountain

Annual herb to 2 ft. tall; leaves 1–3 in. long, toothless, the upper leaves conspicuously bordered with white; "flower" with conspicuous white petal-like appendages. Widely cultivated in gardens and lawns as border plants, it is a native of dry plains and valleys from Montana to Mexico and sometimes escapes in eastern United States. The use of a decoction of this plant in an effort to cause abortion resulted in the death of a young woman.

E. milii Ch. des Moulins (*E. splendens* Hook.)—Crown-of-thorns (Figure 32)

A woody, branched, very spiny, shrublike plant to 4 ft. tall; leaves few and scattered mostly on the new growth, 1–2½

Figure 32. Crown-of-thorns (*Euphorbia milii*) A shrubby, spiny, ornamental plant with milky juice.

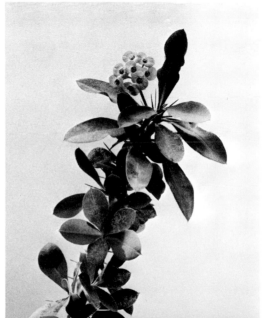

in. long, not toothed; "flowers" located above 2 broad red bracts each about ½ in. across. This attractive shrub is cultivated as a house or patio plant, or very commonly grown outside in southern United States and Hawaii.

E. pulcherrima Willd.—Poinsettia

A shrub with large alternate leaves, blades 3–6 in. long, not toothed or with a few large teeth; "flowers" clustered at the top with red, pink, or cream leaves just below and forming the showy parts of the plant. This is a popular winter-flowering shrub used extensively at Christmas as an indoor ornamental, and planted outside in southern United States and Hawaii as a shrub or hedge.

E. tirucallii L.—Milk bush, Indian tree spurge, pencil tree, Malabar tree, monkey fiddle (Figure 33)

A succulent, spineless, shrublike plant, the branches green and cylindric, about ¼–½ in. thick; leaves linear, small, and only a few limited to the tips of the branches and soon dropping. This rather odd-looking plant is cultivated as a potted plant for the house and patio.

Poisoning: The spurges contain a toxic principle in the milky sap which can cause dermatitis in some people and severe poisoning if eaten in quantity. There are records of death caused by caper spurge and snow-on-the-mountain and severe irritation to the mouth, throat, and stomach by other species. These various spurges are of particular importance since many are very common in lawns or in the home.

To the physician: Gastric lavage or emesis; symptomatic.

Note: It is hearsay that all plants with milky juice are poisonous, for there are a number of harmless and even very edible plants such as lettuce, dandelion, or mulberry with this characteristic. Nevertheless, since many poisonous plants, such as milky-cap mushroom, spurge, dogbane, and milkweed do have milky juice, it should be considered a signal for caution.

Hippomane mancinella L.—Manchineel

The fruit of the manchineel is extremely poisonous if

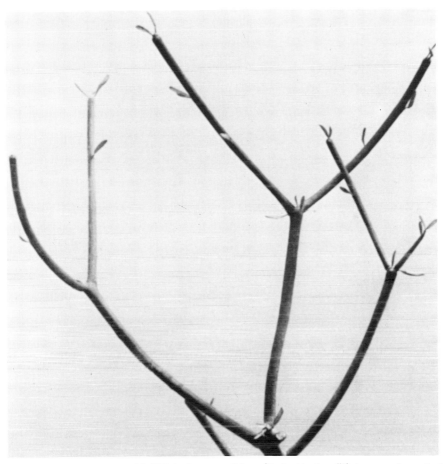

Figure 33. Milk bush or pencil tree (*Euphorbia tirucallii*) An unusual succulent ornamental with milky juice.

eaten, causing stomach pain, vomiting, and bloody diarrhea. See p. 17 for a description of the tree.

To the physician: Gastric lavage or emesis; mineral oil.

Hura crepitans L.—Sandbox tree, monkey dinner bell

This large spiny tree from the American tropics is occasionally planted as an ornamental in southern United States and Hawaii for the curious explosive fruits. The capsules, when ripe, spring open with explosive violence and loud noise and throw the seeds many feet. The milky juice causes severe vomiting and diarrhea when eaten. Two or 3 seeds are sufficient to cause severe symptoms. The bark is used to kill fish in some tropical areas.

To the physician: Gastric lavage or emesis; symptomatic.

Jatropha spp.

Description: Trees and shrubs; leaves alternate, stalked, palmately veined, and 3–5 lobed or deeply cut into 9–11 segments; flowers red or yellow, small; fruit a capsule.

J. curcas L.—Purge nut, curcas bean, physic nut, Barbados nut (Figure 34)

This species is widely cultivated in Florida and Hawaii as an ornamental.

J. gossypifolia L.—Bellyache bush

This is a shrub cultivated as an ornamental in southern Florida and Hawaii.

J. integerrima Jacq.—Peregrina

This species is cultivated as an ornamental in southern Florida.

J. multifida L.—Physic nut, coral plant

Physic nut is a native of tropical regions and is frequently planted from southern Florida to Texas and in Hawaii.

Poisoning: Sap from all parts of the plants contains curcin, a toxalbumin. The attractive fruits or seeds, not infrequently eaten by children, cause nausea, violent vomiting, bloody diarrhea, and coma from a few minutes to several hours after eating. Three seeds are possibly sufficient to cause severe symptoms. It is considered one of the chief causes of poisoning in south Florida.

To the physician: Gastric lavage or emesis; symptomatic; treat for shock.

Manihot esculenta Crantz—Cassava, manioc, tapioca

Cassava, a bushy herb or shrub and native of Brazil, is widely cultivated throughout the tropics for the tuberous edible roots which are used as a starchy food. The underground tubers, similar to sweet potatoes, are boiled and eaten or fixed in various ways such as in the formation of tapioca. There is no real danger as normally used.

The raw root, or peelings of the tubers, however, can form high concentrations of prussic acid sufficient to cause death from cyanide poisoning. The greatest danger lies in the areas of southern United States where the plants are occasionally cultivated and the roots are available to children or to those adults unfamiliar with the correct process of fixing the roots.

To the physician: Immediate gastric lavage or emesis; treat for cyanide poisoning.

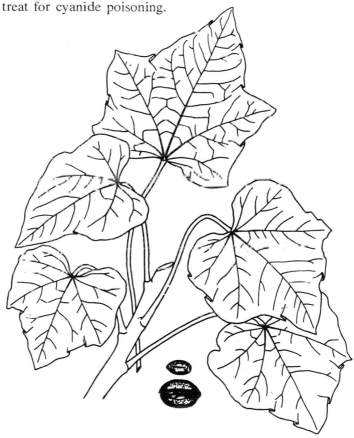

Figure 34. Purge nut or Barbados nut (*Jatropha curcus*) An ornamental of tropical regions with poisonous seeds. Courtesy of the Florida Agricultural Experiment Station.

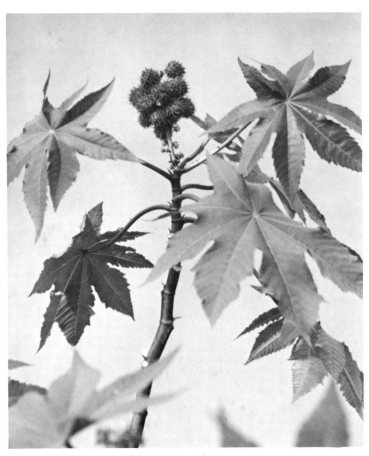

Figure 35. Castor bean (*Ricinus communis*) An attractive ornamental and commercial plant with very dangerous seeds. (See facing page.) Close-up of seeds a USDA Photograph.

Ricinus communis L.—Castor bean, castor-oil plant (Figure 35)

Description: Shrublike herb, stems 4–12 ft. tall, branched, green to reddish or purple; leaves alternate, simple, long-stalked, to 30 in. wide and palmately lobed with 5–11 long lobes which are toothed on the margins, green or reddish; fruits oval, green or red, and covered with fleshy spines; seeds 3 per capsule, about ½–¾ in. across, elliptical, glossy, black or white or usually mottled with gray, black, brown, and white.

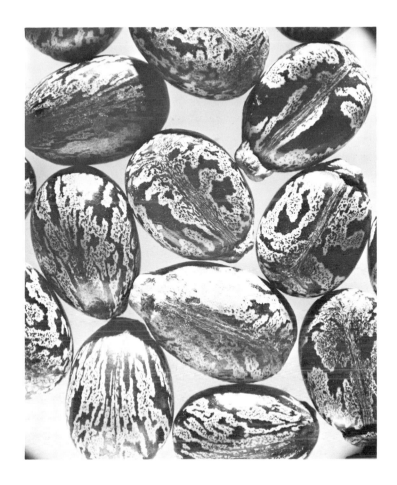

Occurrence: Castor bean is cultivated as an ornamental in yards, and occasionally escapes, mostly in the southern United States and lower altitudes in Hawaii. It is grown commercially in California and southern states for the oil extracted from the seeds.

Poisoning: The seeds, if chewed, are most toxic; leaves are less toxic. Ricin, a phytotoxin, causes burning of the mouth and throat, nausea, vomiting, severe stomach pains, diarrhea, excessive thirst, prostration, dullness of vision, convulsions, uremia, and death. One to 3 seeds can be fatal to a child; 2 to 4 seeds may cause very severe poisoning or fatality in an adult, and 8 are generally fatal to an adult.

Death from uremia may occur up to 12 days after eating. If seeds are swallowed without chewing, poisoning is unlikely because of the hard seed coat.

This is a commonly cultivated plant, and the seeds are readily available for children to play with or for making necklaces. The danger may be eliminated if the flower stalks or seed heads are removed before the fruits are mature. If this is done regularly, castor bean can be a beautiful, and safe, ornamental plant for the yard. Otherwise it is one of the chief causes of poisoning among children.

The seeds are used for the extraction of castor oil, used as a medicinal drug, an ingredient in soaps, and as a lubricant.

To the physician: Immediate gastric lavage or emesis; supportive; keep urine alkaline with 5–15 gm. sodium bicarbonate daily.

HEATH FAMILY—*Ericaceae*

Kalmia latifolia L.—Mountain laurel, mountain ivy, ivy bush (Figure 36)

Description: Large evergreen shrubs to 35 ft. tall; leaves nearly all alternate, 1½–4½ in. long, margin not toothed, bright green below and dark green above; flowers in terminal clusters, white to rose, anthers held in small pockets in the side of the corolla tube until pollination; fruit a dry capsule.

Occurrence: Mountain laurel is found in moist woods and along streams, on mountain tops and in heath balds (laurel slicks) of eastern Canada southward in the Appalachian Mountains and Piedmont and infrequently in the eastern Coastal Plain. This is one of the most beautiful flowering shrubs of the Appalachians. It is the state flower of Connecticut and Pennsylvania.

The related *K. angustifolia* L. and *K. polifolia* Wang., lambkill, sheep laurel, wicky, swamp laurel, are small shrubs with opposite or whorled leaves and narrow inflorescences of small flowers. They occur in wet meadows, bogs, and pocosins from Alaska to California and Colorado and northeastward to eastern Canada and southward in the

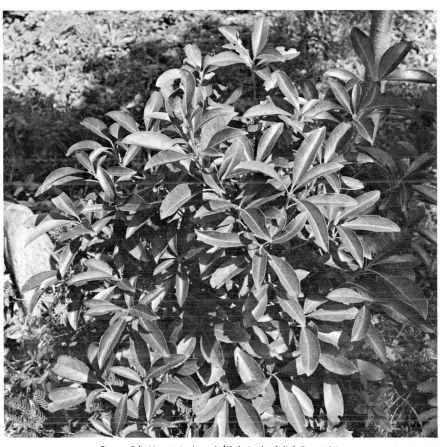

Figure 36. Mountain laurel (*Kalmia latifolia*) Beautiful evergreen shrub with clusters of pink flowers.

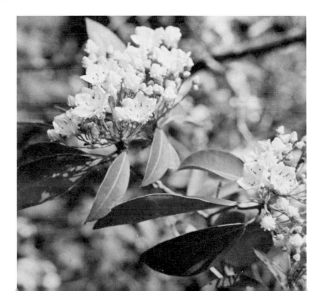

eastern Coastal Plain and bogs of the mountains to South Carolina.

Poisoning: The leaves, twigs, flowers, and pollen grains contain andromedotoxin, which is a toxic resinoid causing watering of the mouth, eyes, and nose, loss of energy, slow pulse, vomiting, low blood pressure, lack of co-ordination, convulsions, and progressive paralysis of arms and legs until death. Poison honey is made occasionally in the mountains when bees visit laurel or rhododendron. The honey is so very bitter and astringent to taste, however, that poisonous amounts would not be eaten. Children have been poisoned by sucking on the flowers and making "tea" from the leaves.

To the physician: Gastric lavage or emesis; activated charcoal; atropine; hypotensive drugs.

Rhododendron spp.—Rhododendron, laurel, rose bay, azalea (Figure 37)

Rhododendrons are evergreen shrubs often forming dense growths in Canada and southward in the Appalachians and the West Coast. The leaves are larger than in *Kalmia* and the larger showy flowers are in globose clusters. *Rhododendron maximum* L. is the most common in the East and is the state flower of West Virginia; *R. macrophyllum* D. Don is common on the West Coast and is the state flower of Washington.

Azaleas are native deciduous shrubs of the United States or evergreen species introduced from Asia and cultivated extensively for the showy flowers.

Poisoning: Rhododendrons and azaleas contain the same toxic principle as found in *Kalmia*. Although cases of poisoning are rare, they should be suspected of possible danger.

OLIVE FAMILY—*Oleaceae*

Ligustrum vulgare L.—Privet, ligustrum, hedge

This deciduous shrub with small opposite leaves is very commonly planted as a hedge or shrub and has escaped cultivation into woods and along creeks throughout the

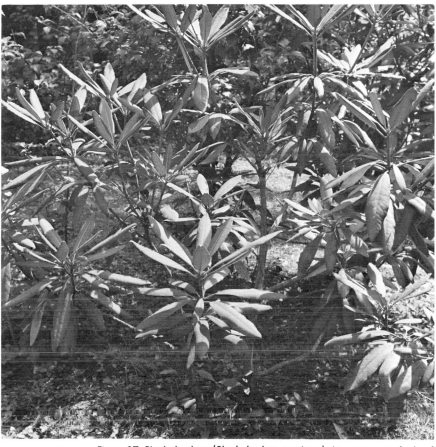

Figure 37. Rhododendron (*Rhododendron maximum*) An evergreen shrub of eastern United States with large clusters of white to pink flowers.

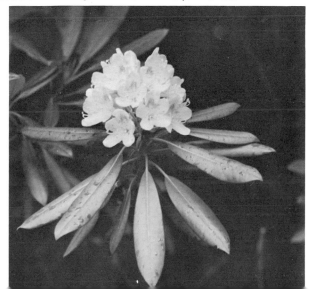

area. The blue or nearly black berries have been the cause of fatal poisoning to children in Europe. Although few cases of poisoning have been recorded for this country, privet should be treated with caution and the fruits kept away from infants. There are a number of species of *Ligustrum* which are deciduous or evergreen and commonly planted.

LOGANIA FAMILY—*Loganiaceae*

Gelsemium sempervirens (L.) Ait. f.—Yellow jessamine, Carolina jessamine (Figure 38)

Description: Woody vine, trailing or high-climbing; leaves opposite, short-stalked, lanceolate, ½–2½ in. long, margin smooth; flowers in early spring, yellow and very aromatic, tubular with 5 petal lobes, 1–1½ in. long; fruit a thin, flattened capsule, less than 1 in. long and with a short beak at the top.

Occurrence: Yellow jessamine is found throughout the southeastern Coastal Plain and eastern Piedmont northward to Virginia; it occurs in woods, on fences, in fields and thickets. It is very common and is one of the most beautiful vines of the early spring in the southeast. It is the state flower of South Carolina. The less common *G. rankinii* Small, in the Coastal Plain from North Carolina to Louisiana, is similar to *G. sempervirens* but is not aromatic. It may also be poisonous.

Poisoning: The alkaloids gelsemine, gelseminine, and gelsemoidine are found throughout the plant, with greatest concentrations in the roots and nectar of the flowers. Children have been severely poisoned by chewing on the leaves and sucking the nectar from the flowers. Honeybees are also poisoned, and a poison honey is occasionally made. Symptoms are profuse sweating, muscular weakness, convulsions, depression, and paralysis of the motor nerve endings. Rootstocks are used as a source of drugs for medicinal purposes.

To the physician: Gastric lavage or emesis; symptomatic; atropine 2 mg. IM as needed; artificial respiration.

The well-known poison strychnine comes from the seeds of *Strychnos nux-vomica* L., also of this family. The flowers

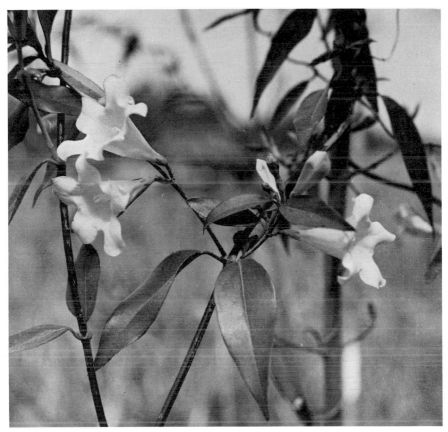

Figure 38. Yellow jessamine (*Gelsemium sempervirens*) A trailing or high-climbing vine with yellow and aromatic flowers.

are also poisonous. It is a native of India and is planted rarely in Hawaii.

DOGBANE FAMILY—*Apocynaceae*

Allamanda cathartica L.—Yellow allamanda (Figure 39)

Description: A woody vine most commonly pruned to a shrub to 15 ft. tall; leaves glossy and leathery, elliptical, 4–6 in. long, opposite or in whorls of 3–4; flowers yellow, aromatic, bell-shaped with 5-petal lobes and a tubular throat, in clusters near the ends of the branches; fruit a prickly capsule.

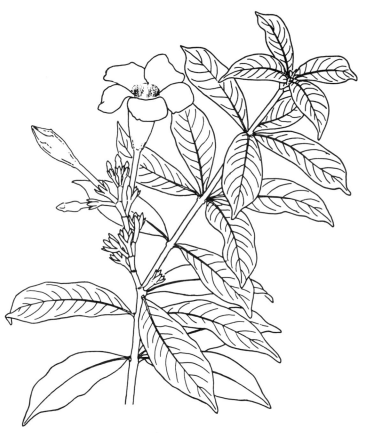

Figure 39. Yellow allamanda (*Allamanda cathartica*) A popular ornamental shrub of the subtropics and tropics with yellow waxy flowers. Courtesy of the Florida Agricultural Experiment Station.

Occurrence: A native of Brazil, yellow allamanda is very commonly cultivated as an ornamental in southern United States and Hawaii.

Poisoning: All parts, but mostly the fruit and cell sap in the stems and leaves, cause a minor stomach upset. The action of the extract, long known by the native tribes of South America, is the basis for the specific epithet *cathartica* named by Linnaeus in 1771.

To the physician: Gastric lavage or emesis; symptomatic.

Apocynum cannabinum L.—Dogbane, Indian hemp (Figure 40)

Description: Perennial herbs with milky juice; leaves

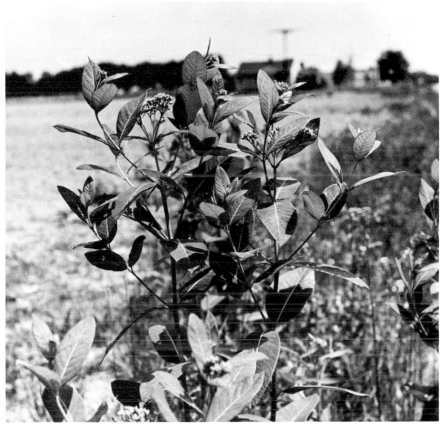

Figure 40. Dogbane (*Apocynum cannabinum*) A common native weed of potential danger to children.

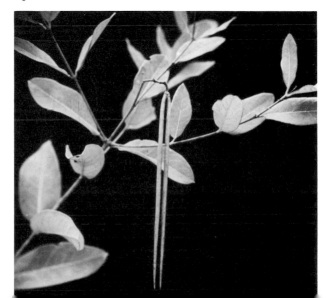

opposite, simple, margins not toothed; flowers small, pink-tinged, appearing in early summer; fruit 2 long and slender follicles containing many seeds with long silky hairs.

Occurrence: Dogbane is a common weed in open fields and pastures, along roadsides, and in waste places throughout the United States and Canada. The related species may also be poisonous.

Poisoning: Although cases of poisoning to humans are not known, dogbane should be suspected since many authorities consider it poisonous to livestock.

Ervatamia coronaria Stapf.—Crape jasmine (Figure 41)

This shrub, a native of India and naturalized in many tropical areas, has waxy white flowers 1½–2 in. across, often double in some forms, and quite fragrant.

It is planted in southern Florida and considered potentially

Figure 41. Crape jasmine (*Ervatamia coronaria*) A potentially poisonous shrub cultivated in the subtropics and tropics. Courtesy of the Florida Agricultural Experiment Station.

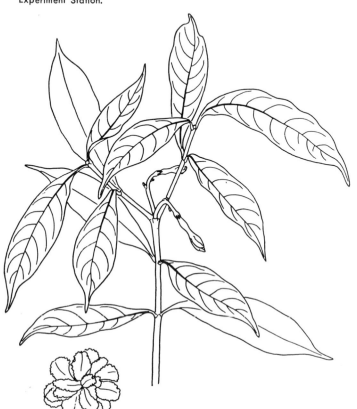

poisonous although no cases have been reported in this country.

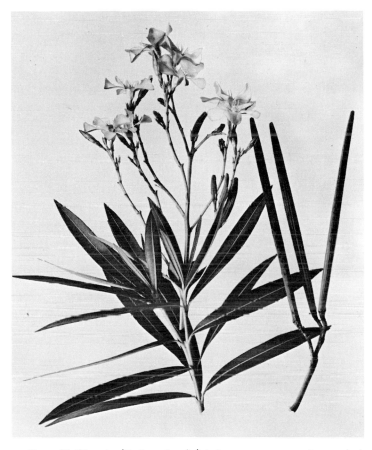

Figure 42. Oleander (*Nerium oleander*) A dangerous evergreen tree or shrub of warm climates.   USDA Photograph.

Nerium oleander L.—Oleander (Figure 42)

Description: An evergreen shrub or small tree to 25 ft. tall, with thick gummy clear sap; leaves short-stalked, opposite or in whorls of 3, narrow, leathery, 3–10 in. long, margins not toothed, veins light yellowish and conspicuous; flowers appearing in summer, in clusters at the tips of the twigs, white to pink to deep red, about 1–3 in. across and sometimes double in certain horticultural forms.

Occurrence: Oleander is a native of southern Europe and has been commonly cultivated as an ornamental in southern United States and California. *N. indicum* Mill. is common in Hawaii.

Poisoning: The twigs, green or dry leaves, and flowers contain cardiac glycosides nerioside and oleandroside. These are extremely poisonous and cause nausea, severe vomiting, stomach pain, dizziness, slowed pulse, irregular heartbeat, marked dilation of pupils, bloody diarrhea, drowsiness, unconsciousness, paralysis of the lungs, and death. A single leaf is said to be sufficient to kill an adult, and severe poisoning has resulted from using the branches as skewers to roast meat over an open fire in Florida; children have been poisoned by chewing the leaves and also by sucking the nectar from the flowers. A poison honey is made by bees visiting the flowers.

To the physician: Gastric lavage or emesis; symptomatic and supportive; potassium, procainamide, quinidine sulfate, disodium salt of edelate (Na_2EDTA) have all been used effectively.

Ochrosia elliptica Labill—Ochrosia plum

A small tree native of New Caledonia, it is grown in Florida and Hawaii for its ornamental foliage and fruits. The bright red, white-fleshed fruits (drupes) are considered poisonous.

Thevetia peruviana Schum.—Yellow oleander, lucky nut, tiger apple, be-still tree

Description: A shrub or tree to 30 ft. tall with a diffusely branched dense crown; leaves alternate, dark green, and glossy, linear, 6 in. long and ¼–½ in. wide; flowers yellow or dull orange, tubular to 3 in. long and with 5 petal lobes, in small clusters at the tips of twigs; fruit a fleshy triangular drupe turning yellow then black.

Occurrence: This attractive shrub, which is native to tropical America, is commonly cultivated as an ornamental in southern United States and Hawaii.

Poisoning: A cardiac glycoside, thevetin, is found throughout the plant but is most concentrated in the fruit. One drupe can cause death, preceded by vomiting, weak pulse, and convulsions. Deaths have been reported in Florida and the Hawaiian Islands. It is considered to be the most frequent cause of poisonings in Hawaii.

To the physician: Gastric lavage or emesis; supportive; atropine.

Urechites spp.—Yellow nightshade, wild allamanda

These are woody vines or shrubs, native of southern Florida, Central America, and the West Indies. The flowers are tubular, somewhat funnel-shaped, 5-parted, and yellow; all parts have milky juice; seed pods (follicles) long and slender.

The follicles cause burning of the mouth and throat, drowsiness, paralysis, convulsions, and heart failure if eaten in quantity.

To the physician: Gastric lavage or emesis; symptomatic.

MILKWEED FAMILY—*Asclepiadaceae*

Cryptostegia grandiflora R. Br.—Rubber vine, purple or pink allamanda

Description: A woody vine with milky sap, often pruned to a shrub; leaves opposite, dark waxy green, leathery, to 5 in. long; flowers purple, funnel-shaped; fruit a sharply angled follicle.

Occurrence: This attractive vine is cultivated as an ornamental in southern United States and Hawaii and has escaped in waste places in those areas.

Poisoning: All parts may cause severe stomach and intestinal upset, and cases of death have been reported from India. The related milkweeds (*Asclepias* spp.) are poisonous to livestock and may be dangerous to children if eaten in quantity. Also the related *Calotropis gigantea* Ait., crownflower, of Hawaii is dangerous.

To the physician: Gastric lavage or emesis; symptomatic.

HONEYSUCKLE FAMILY—*Caprifoliaceae*

Sambucus spp.—Elder, elderberry

Description: Shrubs with soft wood and large pith with long internodes between the opposite, pinnately divided leaves; leaflets 5–11 per leaf, toothed on the margins, deciduous; flowers small, 5-lobed, white, in large terminal clusters; fruit berry-like and juicy, red or black.

S. canadensis L.—Elder, elderberry (Figure 43)

Flowers in flat-topped clusters; fruit purple-black; pith of stem white. This is a very common shrub in woods and low fields and waste places or along ditches from Canada south to Florida and Arizona.

Figure 43. Elderberry (*Sambucus canadensis*) A common shrub with divided leaves and flat-topped clusters of small white flowers. Some parts are edible, some poisonous.

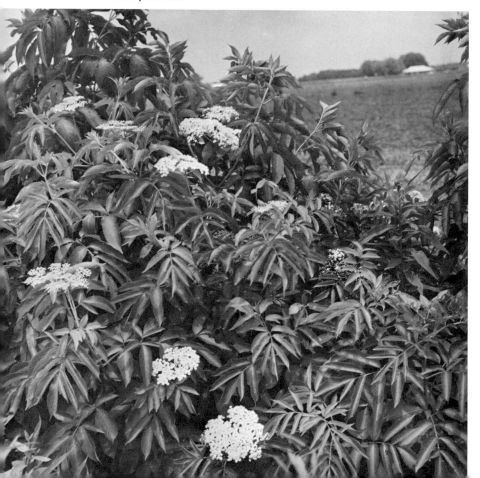

S. mexicana var. *bipinnata* (Schl. & Cham.) Schwerin— Mexican elder

> This variety is the common elder in Hawaii.

S. pubens Michx.—Red-berried elder

> Flowers in ovoid clusters; fruit red; pith of stem brown. This species is fairly common in moist open woods and fields, Alaska to southern California, eastward in Canada, south in the Rockies to Colorado and New Mexico, and into North Carolina and Georgia along the higher elevations of the Appalachians.

S. simpsonii Rehd.—Gulf elder, southern elder

> Similar to *S. canadensis* but the lower leaflets are again pinnately divided. It is a common shrub of roadside ditches, hammocks, and marshes from Florida to Louisiana.
>
> There are other species in western United States and Canada, from the Rockies to the Pacific coast, and in Hawaii. All are potentially dangerous.
>
> Poisoning: The roots, stems, and leaves, and much less the flowers and unripe berries, contain a poisonous alkaloid and cyanogenic glycoside causing nausea, vomiting, and diarrhea. Children have been poisoned by making blowguns, whistles, and popguns out of the stems and having them in their mouths. The flowers and ripe fruit are edible without harm and are frequently used for pies, wine, jelly, and pancakes.
>
> To the physician: Gastric lavage or emesis; treat for cyanide poisoning.

POTATO FAMILY—*Solanaceae*

Atropa belladonna L.—Belladonna, deadly nightshade

> Description: Coarse, branched herb to 5 ft. tall; leaves alternate, simple, ovate and smooth-margined, appearing crowded because of short axillary branches with leaves; flowers dull purple, tubular and about 1 in. long; fruit a purple to black berry with a persistent 5-lobed calyx.
>
> Occurrence: Belladonna is a native of Europe and is planted as a garden ornamental in the United States.

Poisoning: The alkaloid atropine is found throughout the plant (berries, leaves, roots, flowers) but the black berries have been the part usually eaten. Symptoms are fever, rapid heartbeat, dilation of pupils, skin flushed hot and dry. It can be fatal, with as few as 3 berries sufficient to kill a child. Atropine, in correct amounts, is one of the most useful plant drugs.

To the physician: Gastric lavage (4 per cent tannic acid solution) or emesis; pilocarpine for dry mouth and visual disturbance.

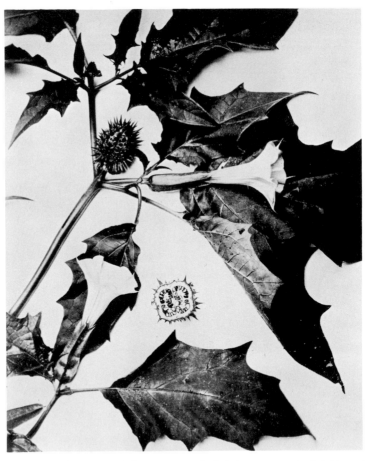

Figure 44. Jimsonweed (*Datura stramonium*) A frequent weed of fields and disturbed areas with white to bluish flowers and prickly fruits. USDA Photograph.

Cestrum spp.—Jessamine, cestrum

> Description: A sprawling shrub to 12 ft. tall; leaves alternate, simple and smooth-margined; flowers tubular, ⅓–1 in. long, greenish white, greenish yellow, or cream; fruit a small berry.

C. diurnum L.—Day-blooming jessamine

> Flowers white and aromatic during the day; berry purple. This is cultivated and has escaped in Florida and Hawaii.

C. nocturnum L.—Night-blooming jessamine, poisonberry

> Flowers greenish white to cream, aromatic at night; berry white. It is cultivated as an ornamental in southern United States and is one of the most common cestrums in Hawaii.

C. parqui L'Her.—Green cestrum, willow-leaved jessamine

> Similar to *C. nocturnum* but the leaves are less than 1 in. wide. It is cultivated as an ornamental and found growing wild in woods and along roadsides from Florida to Texas.
>
> Poisoning: Eating of any part of these plants can result in symptoms resembling atropine poisoning with headache, nausea, dizziness, hallucinations, muscular spasms and nervousness, high temperature, watering of mouth, and paralysis. Cases of poisoning among children and pets are on record.
>
> To the physician: Gastric lavage or emesis; symptomatic.

Datura stramonium L.—Jimsonweed, Jamestown weed, thornapple, stinkweed, datura (Figure 44)

> Description: Large annual to 5 ft. tall, wide-branching near the tip; stem green to purplish, ill-scented; leaves alternate, simple, ovate-elliptic, 3–8 in. long, short-stalked, with irregular large teeth on the margin; flowers funnel-shaped, white to bluish purple; fruit a dry, ovoid capsule covered with many sharp prickles.
>
> Occurrence: Jimsonweed is a very common weed of fields, pastures, gardens, roadsides, and waste places; widespread throughout North and South America and Hawaii.

D. metaloides Dunal

> Found in fields, along roadsides, and on plains from Colorado south to Texas, Mexico, and California.

D. metel L.—Metel, downy thornapple, devil's trumpet

An ornamental shrublike herb of the eastern United States and Hawaii.

D. suaveolens H.&B.—Angel's trumpet (Figure 45)

An ornamental shrub or small tree cultivated in southern United States and Hawaii for the large (to 1 ft. long) trumpet-like white flowers.

Poisoning: All parts, particularly the seeds and leaves, contain the alkaloids hyoscyamine, atropine, and hyoscine (scopolamine). Symptoms are thirst, pupil dilation, dry mouth, redness of skin, headache, hallucinations, nausea, rapid pulse, high blood pressure, delirium, convulsions, coma, and death. Children have been poisoned by sucking nectar from the flowers, eating the seeds or making "tea" from the leaves. Even a very small amount (4–5 grams) of leaves or seeds can be fatal to a child. A family of four was poisoned when seeds of jimsonweed were mistakenly added to homemade soup. The leaves and seeds are used as a source of drugs for medicinal purposes.

Jimsonweed has an interesting place in American history. During the time of the Virginia uprising known as Bacon's Rebellion, which occurred in Jamestown in 1676, the soldiers sent to stop the rebellion unfortunately ate the berries of this plant for lack of other food and became deathly ill. The name "jimsonweed" is therefore a corruption of the older and more meaningful "Jamestown weed."

To the physician: Gastric lavage or emesis; pilocarpine for dry mouth and visual disturbance; symptomatic.

Hyoscyamus niger L.—Black henbane, henbane

Description: Erect annual or biennial herb with coarse, hairy stems 1–5 ft. tall; leaves alternate, simple, oblong with a few coarse teeth, not stalked; flowers in the leaf axils, corolla tubular and 5-lobed, greenish yellow or yellowish with purple veins; fruit a rounded capsule inclosed by a 5-lobed calyx.

Occurrence: Black henbane is cultivated and has escaped along roads, in waste places, and around buildings across

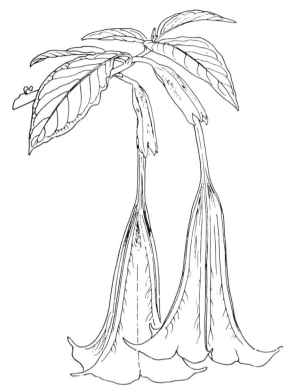

Figure 45. Angel's trumpet (*Datura suaveolens*) An ornamental of subtropical and tropical areas with foot-long tubular flowers. Courtesy of the Florida Agricultural Experiment Station.

southern Canada and northern United States. It is particularly common in the northern Rocky Mountains.

Poisoning: The alkaloids hyoscyamine, hyoscine, and atropine occur throughout the plant and cause watering of mouth, headache, nausea, rapid pulse, convulsions, coma, and death.

To the physician: Gastric lavage (4 per cent tannic acid solution) or emesis; symptomatic and supportive.

Lycopersicon esculentum Mill.—Tomato

The leaves of the common tomato are poisonous, and children have developed severe reactions from making "tea" from the leaves.

The grafting of tomato plants on stock of jimsonweed to produce hardy tomatoes that would be resistent to cold, resulted in severe poisoning in several members of a family in Hawkins County, Tennessee, after they ate the tomatoes.

Nicandra physalodes (L.) Gaertn.—Apple-of-Peru, shoofly plant

This large herb is closely related to *Physalis* and differs by its pale blue (rather than yellow) corolla and dry (rather than juicy) berry. It has been introduced from Peru and has become established, out of cultivation, as an occasional weed in barn lots and fields throughout most of the United States and Hawaii. The poisoning is expected to be similar to that in *Physalis,* although no cases have been reported.

Nicotiana tabacum L.—Tobacco

Aside from the effects from smoking, tobacco leaves have caused severe poisoning when eaten as cooked greens. The related *N. glauca* Graham (tree tobacco) is a shrub or small tree cultivated as an ornamental in Florida and California and is a weed in California and Hawaii. It has been the cause of illness in children sucking the flowers, and death when leaves were chopped up and used in a green salad. *N. trigonophylla* Dunal (wild tobacco) of dry desert soils in southwestern United States caused poisoning and one death in a California family that ate the leaves as boiled greens. Additional species are possibly equally dangerous.

Poisoning: The alkaloid nicotine is extremely poisonous, causing severe vomiting, diarrhea, slow pulse, dizziness, collapse, and respiratory failure.

To the physician: Gastric lavage or emesis; activated charcoal, artificial respiration and oxygen, tannin administered orally.

Physalis spp.—Ground cherry, Jerusalem cherry, Chinese lantern, strawberry tomato

Description: Perennial herbs with erect stem spreading at the top, often much branched; leaves alternate, simple, smooth-margined or irregularly toothed; flowers axillary, nodding, mostly solitary, corolla short, funnel-shaped or bell-shaped, yellowish or yellow-green with a dark center; fruit a globose juicy berry turning yellow and mostly enclosed by the enlarged calyx.

Occurrence: There are a number of species native in pastures, meadows, fields, woods, and roadsides throughout the United States. Some types are cultivated as ornamentals. *P. peruviana* L. is common in Hawaii and is used for jelly and preserves.

Poisoning: The leaves and *unripe* fruit are poisonous.

To the physician: Gastric lavage or emesis; symptomatic.

Solandra spp.—Trumpet flower, chalice vine

These very large funnel- to bell-shaped, showy, white or yellow flowers are cultivated as house plants or outside in southern United States and Hawaii.

Poisoning is similar to that in *Solanum* and has resulted from children eating the leaves and flowers.

Solanum spp.—Nightshade

Description: Herbs or shrublike plants with simple alternate leaves; flowers with calyx and corolla 5-lobed and wide-spreading, the large yellow anthers erect and conspicuous; fruit a berry.

S. americanum Miller and *S. nigrum* L.—Nightshade, black nightshade (Figure 46)

Annual branched herbs with dark dull green leaves, ovate or lanceolate, toothless to slightly toothed on the margins; flowers small and white; fruit black when ripe, glossy and in an umbel (*S. americanum*) or dull and in a raceme (*S. nigrum*). *S. americanum* is a common native weed of waste places, old fields, ditches, and roadsides, fence rows, or edges of woods throughout the United States. The European *S. nigrum* is established as a weed in similar habitats in the United States and Hawaii.

S. carolinense L.—Horse nettle, wild tomato (Figure 47)

This is a very common prickly weed throughout the United States. The yellow berries are conspicuous and sometimes used as a source of drugs for medicinal purposes. A child died a few years ago in Philadelphia from eating the berries.

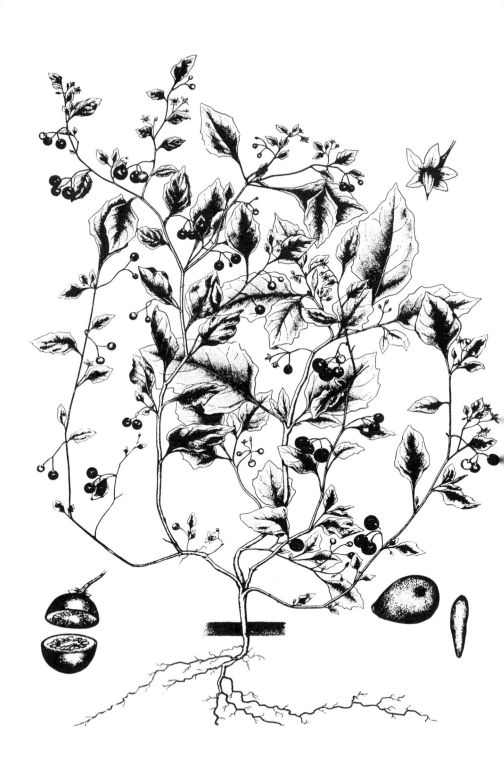

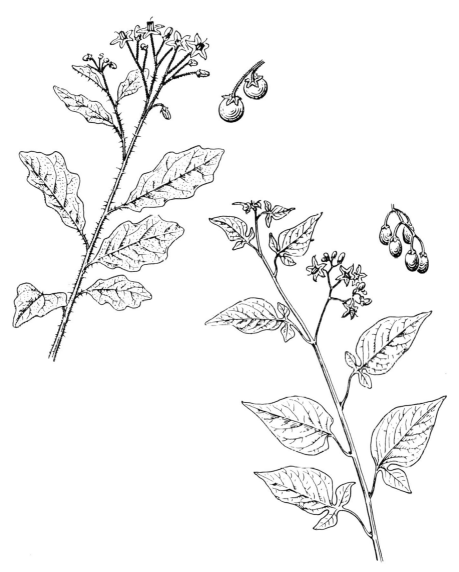

Figure 46. Black nightshade (*Solanum americanum*) A native weed with shiny black berries. Drawing a USDA Photograph. (See facing page.)

Figure 47. Horse nettle (*Solanum carolinense*) A common prickly weed with yellow berries. From *Flora of West Virginia*, courtesy of Dr. E. L. Core.

Figure 48. Deadly nightshade (*Solanum dulcamara*) An attractive woody plant with purple flowers and red berries. From *Flora of West Virginia*, courtesy of of Dr. E. L. Core.

S. dulcamara L.—Deadly nightshade, climbing nightshade, European bittersweet (Figure 48)

A woody vine or shrub with purple flowers and red berries. It is a native of Eurasia and has become naturalized on moist stream or pond banks and in low damp woods from Canada to California, Kansas, Tennessee, and North Carolina.

S. pseudocapsicum L.—Jerusalem cherry

Growing wild in Hawaii or as an ornamental potted plant throughout the United States, this species is prized for its bright red berries.

S. sodomeum L.—Apple of Sodom, yellow-fruited popolo

This is a common weed in Hawaii. It is a prickly shrub with blue flowers.

S. tuberosum L.—Potato, irish potato, white potato

This common vegetable is grown throughout the area and only rarely escapes cultivation.

All other species of *Solanum* should be suspected of being poisonous.

Poisoning: Solanine, a glyco-alkaloid, is found throughout the plant, with the highest concentrations in the unripened fruit. Symptoms are stomach pain, lower temperature, paralysis, dilated pupils, vomiting, diarrhea, shock, circulatory and respiratory depression, loss of sensation, and death. Solanine is extremely toxic and small amounts can be deadly.

Misconceptions occur concerning the poisonous qualities of the solanums, probably because of the harmless nature of the completely ripe fruit of certain species. Many are considered edible. However, cases of poisoning from eating the *unripened* fruits have been reported from the Hawaiian Islands and North America. Children have been poisoned from black nightshade, deadly nightshade, and horse nettle. Green and spoiled potatoes, and potato sprouts have caused severe cases of poisoning. Never eat potato tubers if they look spoiled or green below the skin, and always discard the sprouts.

To the physician: Gastric lavage or emesis; symptomatic; support respiration, paraldehyde (2–10 ml. IM).

SNAPDRAGON FAMILY—*Scrophulariaceae*

Digitalis purpurea L.—Foxglove

Description: Biennial herb with alternate, simple, toothed leaves; flowers in a showy terminal raceme, tubular to 3 in. long, pendent, purple, pink, rose, yellow, or white and spotted on the inside bottom of the tube; fruit a dry capsule.

Occurrence: Foxglove is a native of Europe and is commonly planted in the United States and Hawaii as a garden ornamental. It is naturalized and locally abundant in cleared lands in western United States.

Poisoning: Foxglove has long been known as a source of cardiac or steroid glycosides, some commonly used today for medicinal purposes. Poisoning in adults results mostly from overdoses of the drug digitalis, or much more rarely in children from sucking the flowers or eating the leaves or seeds. Symptoms include nausea, diarrhea, stomach pain, severe headache, irregular heartbeat and pulse, tremors, convulsions, and death.

To the physician: Gastric lavage or emesis; supportive; atropine, potassium, procainamide, quinidine sulfate, disodium salt of edelate (Na_2EDTA) have all been used effectively.

VERVAIN FAMILY—*Verbenaceae*

Duranta repens L.—Golden dewdrop, pigeonberry, duranta, sky-flower

Description: Drooping shrub to 18 ft. tall with stems trailing and often thorny; leaves opposite, rounded, coarsely toothed, to 4 in. long; flowers lilac-blue with yellow eye, to ½ in. across; fruit yellow-orange, to ½ in. across, an 8-seeded berry inclosed by the calyx, in a drooping raceme.

Occurrence: Duranta is a native of tropical America and is cultivated in southern United States and Hawaii as an ornamental shrub or for hedges. It is especially attractive when loaded with masses of yellow-orange berries. Certain horticultural forms have larger flowers or of different colors.

Poisoning: The berries contain a saponin causing drowsiness, fever, and convulsions. Deaths of children from eating the berries are on record.

To the physician: Gastric lavage or emesis; symptomatic.

Lantana camara L.—Lantana, red sage (Figure 49)

Description: Perennial shrub with square twigs and a few scattered spines; leaves simple, opposite or whorled, with toothed margins, ovate, 1–5 in. long; inflorescence a flat-topped cluster of small flowers 1–2 in. across and on a long stalk; flowers small and tubular, 4-parted, white, yellow, or pink changing to orange or red; fruit a drupe, greenish and becoming blue-black when ripe, about ¼–⅜ in. across, fleshy.

Occurrence: Lantana is cultivated as an ornamental shrub in pots or porches or patios in the northern United States and Canada, or as a lawn shrub in the southeastern Coastal Plain, Texas, California, and Hawaii. It is a native of dry woods in the southeastern United States and has escaped cultivation and become weedy in some areas. It is considered to be one of the chief causes of poisoning in Florida.

Poisoning: The fruit contains an alkaloid lantanin or lantadene A. The green, unripened fruit is the most dangerous. Symptoms are stomach and intestinal irritation, muscular, weakness, circulatory collapse, and death. Acute symptoms resemble atropine poisoning. All species are suspected of poisoning.

To the physician: Gastric lavage or emesis; symptomatic and supportive.

LOBELIA FAMILY—*Lobeliaceae*

Lobelia spp.—Lobelia, Indian tobacco, cardinal flower

Description: Herbs with alternate, simple leaves; flowers in a terminal raceme, corolla white, blue, or red, tubular and 2-lipped, with 2 lobes forming the upper lip and 3 forming the lower; fruit a capsule.

Occurrence: There are numerous species of lobelia native in fields, woods, and roadsides throughout the United States.

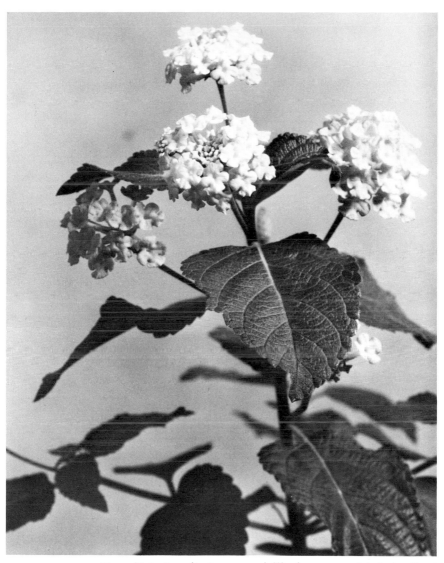

Figure 49. Lantana (*Lantana camara*) Weed or ornamental shrub with attractive yellow, orange, or red flowers and blue-black berries. USDA Photograph.

Poisoning: All parts of the plant contain the alkaloids lobelamine, lobeline, and others. Symptoms include nausea, progressive vomiting, exhaustion and weakness, prostration, stupor, tremors, convulsions, coma, and death. Most cases of human poisoning have resulted from overdoses of a home-made medicinal preparation from *L. inflata* L. (Indian tobacco), which is sometimes used as a commercial source of a medicinal drug.

To the physician: Gastric lavage or emesis; artificial respiration; atropine 2 mg. IM as needed.

ASTER FAMILY—*Asteraceae, Compositae*

Arnica montana L.—Leopard's-bane, mountain tobacco, mountain snuff, arnica root

Description: Perennial, erect herb to 2 ft. tall, unbranched or slightly branched, hairy; basal leaves clustered, 2–5 in. long, stem leaves opposite, few and smaller; flower heads deep yellow, solitary or 3–4 in a cluster, each 2–3 in. across; fruit a small achene.

Occurrence: A native of Europe, arnica is occasionally cultivated in rock gardens or borders of flower beds in northern United States and Canada.

Poisoning: The extract of this European plant is used in medicine, but the flowers and roots have caused vomiting, drowsiness, and coma when eaten by children.

To the physician: Gastric lavage or emesis; symptomatic.

Eupatorium rugosum Houtt.—White snakeroot, fall poison (Figure 50)

Description: Perennial herb to 4 ft. tall with opposit leaves which are ovate, long-stalked, and coarsely toothed on the margins; flowers small, white, in small heads which are arranged in rounded clusters at the top of the plant; fruit a small achene.

Occurrence: White snakeroot is a showy weed of road-sides, fields, open woods, and pastures from Canada southward to Georgia, eastern Texas, and Minnesota; common in the Appalachians and upper Midwest, less frequent in the Piedmont and eastern Coastal Plain.

Poisoning: The entire plant contains tremetol, a complex alcohol, and certain glycosides. A common condition in early colonial times, called "milk sickness," became one of

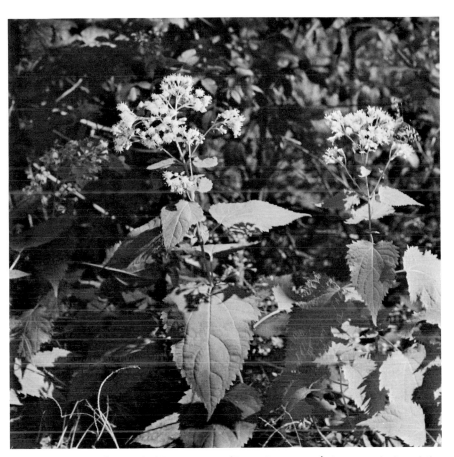

Figure 50. White snakeroot (*Eupatorium rugosum*) A common herb and the cause of "milk sickness" in eastern United States.

the most important causes of human death, reaching its peak during the early 1800's. The greatest number of recorded cases were in North Carolina, Illinois, Indiana, and Ohio. There is a "Milk-sick Ridge" in western North Carolina which attests to the difficulties of those times. This illness was caused by the cows eating white snakeroot so that the poisonous chemical was concentrated in the milk. Symptoms resulting from drinking this poisonous milk included weakness, nausea, severe vomiting, tremors, jaundice, constipation, prostration, delirium, and death.

With processed milk, the condition is now rare, the only danger occurring when raw milk is used from the family cow.

To the physician: Symptomatic; treat for liver damage and anuria.

Haplopappus heterophyllus (Gray) Blake—Rayless goldenrod, jimmy weed, burrow weed

Description: Erect bushy plant 2–4 ft. tall; leaves alternate, slender, and sticky; flowers yellow, in many small heads of 7–15 flowers, clustered at the tips of the stems.

Occurrence: Rayless goldenrod is common in fields or ranges, around watering sites, and along stream banks from Kansas, Oklahoma, and Texas to Colorado, New Mexico, Arizona, and into Mexico. Other species of *Haplopappus* may be equally dangerous.

Poisoning: Like *Eupatorium rugosum,* tremetol is present throughout the plant and similar milk sickness has been a problem in sections of the southwestern United States.

To the physician: Gastric lavage or emesis; symptomatic; treat for liver damage and anuria.

Poisonous and non-poisonous berries

The list which follows includes many native and cultivated berries in the United States and Canada which are often eaten, particularly by children. These are listed here so that one can find out quickly whether a particular kind is poisonous or safe. Although poisonous berries account for many of the cases of poisoning in children, the vast majority of the different kinds are edible. All fleshy fruits (berries, drupes, and pomes) are included under the commonly used term "berry."

It is probably safest to teach children to eat only plants served to them, yet we would never want to deprive any child of the joys of gathering and eating wild fruits. Extensive berry picking should be limited, however, to the commonly eaten types such as strawberry, blackberry, dewberry, red and black raspberry, cranberry, gooseberry, blueberry, huckleberry, citrus, persimmon, pawpaw, plum, apple, and grape. All of these are perfectly safe.

Many berries have long been looked upon with suspicion or thought of as poisonous, perhaps through folklore or because they just look poisonous. However, many of these are edible, in the sense of being nonpoisonous, although sometimes not very palatable. In a few cases some of our common berries are unclassified as to their poisonous or edible nature and should be treated with caution. *Never eat large quantities of an unknown berry.*

Remember that birds, squirrels, and pets often can eat many poisonous fruits without harm, so do not trust what you see them eat. Also keep in mind that it takes fewer berries to poison a child than an adult.

Some of the common uses are given under "Notes on Edibility." For more information see Fernald and Kinsey (1958), Gillespie (1959), Harrington (1967), Heller (1953), Morton (1962), and others on edible plants.

NOTES ON EDIBILITY OF BERRIES

Achras spp.—Sapodilla, dilly: Raw, only when fully ripe

Actaea spp.—Baneberry: *Poisonous,* see pp. 44–46

Akebia quinata—Akebia: Raw

Aleurites spp.—Tung nut, candlenut: *Poisonous,* see pp. 89–90

Amelanchier spp.—Serviceberry, shadberry: Raw, pies, pudding, jelly

Ampelopsis spp.—Ampelopsis, cissus: Unknown, caution!

Anacardium occidentale—Cashew apple: Raw, jelly, preserves

Annona spp.—Custard apple, pond apple, sweetsop, soursop, cherimoya: Raw, jelly

Aralia spp.—Sarsaparilla, Hercules' club, spikenard: Jelly; *poisonous* if raw, see p. 83

Arctostaphylos spp.—Bearberry, kinnikinik, manzanita: Raw, jelly, cider, cooked

Ardisia escallonioides—Marlberry, dogberry: Raw, but not good

Areca catechu—Betel nut: *Poisonous,* see p. 42 see p. 42
Arecastrum romanzoffianum—Queen palm: Caution!
Arisaema triphyllum—Jack-in-the-pulpit: Raw, but peppery
Aronia spp.—Chokeberry: Jelly
Artabotrys uncinatus—Ylang-ylang: Inedible, but not poisonous
Artocarpus spp.—Breadfruit, jackfruit, jakfruit: Raw, jelly, dried
Asimina spp.—Pawpaw, dog apple: Raw, pies, caution!
Asparagus officinalis—Asparagus: Caution!
Atropa belladonna—Belladonna: *Poisonous,* see pp. 111–112 see pp. 111–112
Averrhoa carambola—Carambola: Raw, jelly, drink

Belamcanda chinensis—Blackberry lily: Caution!
Berberis spp.—Barberry: Raw, wine, jelly, pies
Berchemia scandens—Supplejack: Caution!
Blighia sapida—Akee: Caution! see p. 78 see p. 78
Bourreria ovata—Bahama strongbark, strongbark: Raw, but not good
Bumelia spp.—Buckthorn, blackhaw, saffron plum: Raw
Byrsonima lucidum—Locust berry: Raw, but "soapy" taste

Calla palustris—Wild calla: Dried
Callicarpa americana—Beautybush, French mulberry: Raw, but not good
Calocarpum sapota—Red sapote: Raw, jam
Calophyllum inophyllum—Mast-wood: Caution!
Cananga odorata—Lanalana: Raw, but not good
Capsicum frutescens—Chili pepper: Caution!
Carica papaya—Papaya: Raw or cooked
Carissa grandiflora—Natal plum, carissa: Raw, jelly, preserves, sauce
Caryota spp.—Fishtail palm: Caution!
Casasia clusiaefolia—Seven-year apple: Raw fruit pulp
Caulophyllum thalictroides—Blue cohosh: *Poisonous,* see p. 48 see p. 48
Celastrus scandens—Bittersweet: *Poisonous,* see p. 74 see p. 74
Celtis spp.—Hackberry, sugarberry: Raw but astringent
Cephalocereus spp.—Tree cactus: Raw, only when ripe

Cestrum spp.—Jessamines: *Poisonous, see* p. 113

Chaenomeles spp.—Flowering quince: Jelly, jam

Chenopodium capitatum—Strawberry blite: Raw, cooked

Chionanthus virginicus—Fringe tree, old man's beard: Unknown

Chrysobalanus spp.—Cocoplum, gopher apple, ground oak: Raw, jelly

Chrysophyllum spp.—Olive plum, satin leaf, star apple: Raw, jelly

Citharexylum fruticosum—Florida fiddlewood: Raw, but not good

Citrus aurantifolia—Key lime, lime: Juice, pies

Citrus aurantium—Sour orange, Seville orange: Juice, marmalade

Citrus spp.—Orange, lemon, grapefruit: Raw, marmalade, juice

Citrus trifoliatus—Trifoliate orange: Very sour

Clintonia borealis—Clintonia: Unknown, caution!

Clusia rosea—Pitch apple: Caution!

Coccoloba spp.—Sea grape, shore grape, pigeon plum: Raw, jelly, juice, wine

Coccothrinax argentata—Silver palm, thatch palm: Raw, but not good

Cocculus spp.—Moonseed: Caution! may be poisonous

Cocos nucifera—Coconut palm: Raw, cooked

Comandra spp.—Bastard toadflax: Caution!

Cordia sebestena—Scarlet cordia, geiger tree: Raw, if ripe

Cornus spp.—Dogwood, bunchberry: Raw, cooked

Cotoneaster spp.—Cotoneaster: Unknown

Crataegus spp.—Hawthorn: Raw, jelly

Cycas circinalis—Cycad, false sago palm: *Poisonous, see* p. 34

Cydonia oblonga—Quince: Jelly

Daphne mezereum—Daphne: *Poisonous, see* pp. 72–73

Diospyros spp.—Persimmon, black sapote: Raw, pies, pudding—when ripe

Diphylleia cymosa—Umbrella leaf: Caution!

Disporum spp.—Disporum, yellow mandarin: Caution!

Dovyalis spp.—Kei-apple, ketembilla: Jelly, preserves

Duchesnea indica—Indian strawberry: Raw, but not good
Duranta repens—Pigeonberry: *Poisonous, see pp.* 121–122

Elaeagnus spp.—Oleaster, silverberry, Russian olive: Jelly
Empetrum spp.—Crowberry, curlewberry: Raw, pies, jelly
Ephedra spp.—Ephedra: Caution!
Eriobotrya japonica—Loquat, Japan plum: Raw, jelly
Eugenia spp.—Surinam cherry, white stopper, Java plum: Raw, jelly
Euonymus spp.—Strawberry bush: *Poisonous, see p.* 74

Feijoa sellowiana—Guarsteen, pineapple-guava: Raw, jam
Ficus spp.—Fig: Raw, preserves
Flacourtia indica—Ramontchi: Jelly
Forestiera spp.—Wild olive: Caution!
Fortunella spp.—Kumquat: Raw, but acid
Fragaria spp.—Strawberry: Raw, jelly, pies, preserves

Gaultheria spp.—Moxieplum, teaberry, wintergreen, salal: Raw
Gaylussacia spp.—Huckleberry, crackberry: Raw, jelly, pies
Ginkgo biloba—Ginkgo, maidenhair tree: Raw (kernel, not outside)

Harrisia spp.—Apple cactus, prickly apple: Raw
Hedera helix—English ivy: *Poisonous, see pp.* 83–84
Heteromeles arbutifolia—Christmas berry: Raw, cooked, wine
Hippomane mancinella—Manchineel: *Poisonous, see pp.* 92–93
Hylocereus undatus—Night-blooming cereus, pitaya: Raw

Ilex spp.—Holly: Caution! see p. 74

Jatropha spp.—Purge nut: *Poisonous, see pp.* 94–95
Juniperus spp.—Juniper, cedar: Used for flavoring

Karwinskia humboldtiana—Coyotillo: *Poisonous, see p.* 75

Lantana spp.—Lantana: *Poisonous, see pp.* 122–123
Ligustrum spp.—Privet: Caution! see pp. 100, 102
Lindera benzoin—Spicebush, benzoin: Dried for tea

Linum spp.—Flax: Cooked
Liriope spp.—Lily turf: Caution!
Litchi sinesis—Litchi, lychee: Raw, dried (litchi nuts)
Lonicera spp.—Honeysuckle, waterberry: Raw, but not good
Lucuma nervosa—Eggfruit, canistel: Raw
Lycium spp.—Matrimony vine, box-thorn: Caution!

Mahonia spp.—Mahonia, Oregon holly: Unknown, caution!
Maianthemum canadense—Wild lily-of-the-valley: Caution!
Malpighia glabra—Barbados cherry: Jam
Malus spp.—Apple, crab apple: Raw, jelly, pies
Mammea americana—Mammee apple, mamey: Jelly, preserves
Mangifera indica—Mango: Raw, jelly, stewed
Medeola virginiana—Indian cucumber: Unknown, caution!
Melia azedarach—Chinaberry: *Poisonous,* see pp. 77–78
Melicocca bijuga—Spanish lime, mamoncillo: Raw
Melothria pendula—Creeping cucumber, melonette: Raw, but strong laxative
Menispermum canadense—Moonseed: *Poisonous,* see pp. 43–44
Metopium toxiferum—Poisonwood: *Poisonous,* see p. 18
Mitchella repens—Partridgeberry: Raw, but dry
Momordica charantia—Balsam pear: *Poisonous,* see pp. 88–89
Monstera deliciosa—Ceriman, monstera: Raw, if fully ripe
Morus spp.—Mulberry: Raw, pies, jelly—if ripe
Myrtus communis—Myrtle: Raw, flavoring

Nandina domestica—Nandina: Unknown
Nicandra physalodes—Apple-of-Peru: *Poisonous,* see p. 116
Nyssa spp.—Sour gum, black gum, tupelo: Raw, but acrid

Ochrosia elliptica—Ochrosia plum: *Poisonous,* see p. 108
Opuntia spp.—Opuntia cactus, prickly pear: Raw or cooked, jelly
Osmanthus spp.—Osmanthus, devilwood: Unknown

Panax quinquefolia—Ginseng: Raw, but not good
Parthenocissus quinquefolia—Virginia creeper: *Poisonous,* see pp. 75–76

Passiflora spp.—Passion fruit, maypop: Raw, drink
Peltandra virginica—Arrow arum, green arrow: Dried, boiled
Peraphyllum ramosissimum—Squaw apple: Raw, jelly
Persea americana—Avocado: Raw, when ripe
Persea borbonia—Redbay, sweetbay: Raw, but not good
Phorodendron serotinum—Mistletoe: *Poisonous,* see pp. 76–77
Photinia spp.—Christmas berry: Unknown
Phyllanthus acidus—Otaheite gooseberry: Pies, preserves
Physalis spp.—Ground cherry, husk tomato: Jelly if ripe, see pp. 116–117
Phytolacca spp.—Pokeberry: Pies if ripe, see pp. 50–54
Podophyllum peltatum—Mayapple, mandrake: Raw, jelly if ripe, see pp. 47–48
Polygonatum spp.—Soloman's seal: Caution!
Pometia pinnata—Langsir: Roasted
Poncirus trifoliata—Trifoliate orange: Not good, sour
Pontederia cordata—Pickerelweed, pikeweed: Raw, boiled, dried
Prunus spp.—Cherry, plum, peach: Pulp only, see pp. 60-61
Psidium guajava—Guava: Raw, jelly, paste
Punica granatum—Pomegranate: Raw, drink
Pyracantha spp.—Pyracantha, firethorn: Raw, but not good
Pyrularia pubera—Buffalo nut: Caution!
Pyrus spp.—Pear: Raw, jelly

Reynosia septentrionalis—Darling plum: Raw or cooked
Rhacoma spp.—Rhacoma, Christmas berry: Raw
Rhamnus spp.—Buckthorn, cascara: Caution! see p. 75
Rhodomyrtus spp.—Downy myrtle, finger cherry: Caution! see p. 73
Rhus spp. (not *Toxicodendron*)—Sumac: Tea
Ribes spp.—Currant, gooseberry: Raw, jelly
Rivina humilis—Rouge plant: Caution!
Rosa spp.—Rose, rose hip: Raw, jelly
Roystonea spp.—Royal palm: Raw, when ripe
Rubus spp.—Thimbleberry, juneberry, loganberry, blackberry, boysenberry, raspberry, dewberry, nagoonberry, cloudberry, salmonberry, wineberry: Raw, jelly, pies, wine

Sabal palmetto—Cabbage palm, palmetto palm: Raw, syrup
—when ripe

Sambucus spp.—Elderberry: Raw, wine, jelly—only when
ripe, see pp. 110–111

Sapindus spp.—Soapberry: Caution!

Sassafras albidum—Sassafras: Not good

Schinus terebinthifolius—Christmas berry: Caution!

Serenoa repens—Saw palmetto: Not good

Shepherdia spp.—Soapberry, buffalo berry, bullberry: Raw,
jelly, drink

Sideroxylon foetidissimum—False mastic, jungle plum: Raw,
but acid and bitter

Smilacina racemosa—False Solomon's seal, scurvyberry:
Smilacina racemosa—False Solomon's seal, scurvyberr:
Caution!

Smilax spp.—Smilax, greenbrier, carrion flower: Raw

Solanum spp.—Nightshade: *Poisonous,* see pp. 117 120

Sorbus spp.—Mountain ash: Raw, when fully ripe

Spondias spp.—Hogplum, wi tree, vi apple: Raw, preserves

Streptopus spp.—Twisted stalk, Mandarin, liverberry,
scootberry, wild cucumber: Caution!

Strychnos nux-vomica—Strychnine: *Poisonous,* see p. 102

Symphoricarpos spp.—Snowberry, waxberry: Caution!

Symplocos tinctoria—Sweetleaf, horsesugar: Not good

Taxus spp.—Yew, ground hemlock: Raw aril; seed *poisonous,*
see pp. 34–35

Thevetia peruviana—Tiger apple: *Poisonous,* see pp. 108–
109

Torreya spp.—Torreya, stinking cedar: Caution!

Toxicodendron spp.—Poison ivy, oak, and sumac: *Poisonous,*
see pp. 18–22

Trillium spp.—Trillium, wake-robin: Unknown

Triosteum spp.—Wild coffee, feverwort, tinker's weed, horse
gentian: Dried, roasted, drink

Umbellularia californica—California laurel, California bay:
Raw, roasted

Vaccinium spp.—Blueberry, cranberry, sparkleberry: Raw,
jelly, pies

Viburnum spp.—Hobblebush, haw, wild raisin, arrowwood, nannyberry, squashberry: Raw, jelly, pies

Vitis spp.—Grape: Raw, jelly, wine

Waldsteinia fragarioides—Barren strawberry: Raw, but not good

Washingtonia filifera—Washington palm, fan palm: Raw, roasted

Wikstroemia spp.—Akia: Caution!

Ximenia americana—Tallowwood plum, hog plum: Raw, but caution!

Zamia spp.—Coontie, Florida arrowroot: *Poisonous,* see p. 34

Zizyphus jujuba—Jujube: Raw, dried, candied, jam

Zizyphus mauritiana—Indian jujube: Jelly, preserves

POISONING OF PETS

Questions concerning the poisoning of pets are so frequent that the subject should be mentioned briefly. With the animal population exploding just as is the human population, it is not surprising that poisoning of pets is increasing and often presents a serious and complex diagnostic and therapeutic problem for the veterinarian. Coupled with the increased numbers of pets and adding to the potential poisonings is the greater use of exotic plants in and around the home, some of which are poisonous to humans and pets alike.

The great majority of poisoning in pets results from their taking the toxic material in food and water, although occasionally poisoning may result from absorption through a wound or even the unbroken skin. Malicious poisoning is most frequently carried out against dogs and cats, although livestock are sometimes involved. The use of various chemicals to control rabbits, foxes, rats, mice, etc. is common practice, and domesticated animals can be poisoned easily by this bait or even by eating the sick or dead vermin that have eaten the poison. Accidental poisoning may also occur from various substances carelessly left out and available for pets as well as children: chemical dips, dusts and sprays, kerosene, fumigants, soil sterilants, fertilizers, fungicides, herbicides, expended clay pigeons, discarded storage batteries, and many others.

Poisoning of pets by native and cultivated plants is often overlooked and usually dismissed by many people since dogs and cats are primarily meat-eaters. This is a mistake, for while it is true that approximately 90 per cent of their diet is meat, the remaining 10 per cent can be almost anything, including poisonous plants. If eaten in sufficient quantity, most plants poisonous to humans and livestock will also be toxic to dogs and cats and other pets. Cases of such poisoning are fairly common.

Pet birds such as canaries have been poisoned by various fruits or seeds of native and cultivated plants around the home. Dogs have been poisoned by mushrooms, fruits such as balsam pear and nightshade, and bulbs of hyacinth and narcissus. Cats have been poisoned by eating English ivy, and the increased popularity of philodendrons in the home has caused a parallel increase in serious illnesses and numerous deaths among cats by this plant.

Proper care of pets should include a realization of the potential poisoning by plants around the home.

GLOSSARY

ACHENE: A small dry indehiscent one-seeded fruit.

ALTERNATE: Leaf arrangement when only one leaf is at any one level on the stem (Figure 52).

ANNUAL: A plant completing its entire life cycle in one growing season and dying back in the winter.

ANTHER: Pollen sac, on the stamen of a flower (Figure 55).

ARIL: A fleshy or pulpy outer covering of a seed, or an appendage of a seed.

AXIL: The upper angle that a leaf stalk or petiole makes with the stem that bears it.

BERRY: A type of fruit which is usually more or less fleshy throughout.

BIENNIAL: A plant which requires two years to complete its life cycle. The first year's growth is generally vegetative only.

BLADE: The broad and flattened portion of a leaf (Figure 53).

BRACT: A much-reduced leaf, the small scalelike leaves associated with the flowers, or a highly modified leaf associated with flower clusters.

CALYX: A collective term for the sepals of a flower (Figure 55).

CAP: The expanded top of a mushroom (Figure 51).

CAPSULE: A type of fruit which is dry, splits along two or more lines, and has more than one row of seeds.

COMA: A condition of insensibility.

CONVULSION: A violent uncontrolled series of muscular contractions.

COROLLA: A collective term for the petals of a flower (Figure 55).

DELIRIUM: A state of frenzied excitement.

DIARRHEA: Abnormal and frequent discharge of liquid stools from the intestines.

DILATION OF PUPILS: Enlargement of the pupils in the eyes.

DRUPE: A fruit type with a fleshy outside and a stony pit enclosing the seed.

EMETIC: A chemical or substance that causes vomiting, such as syrup of ipecac, a strong solution of table salt, a strong solution of prepared mustard, or strong soapy water.

FOLLICLE: A type of fruit which is dry and opens along only one side.

GILLS: Platelike structures on the bottom of the cap, bearing spores in a mushroom (Figure 51).

GLABROUS: Not hairy.

GLOBOSE: Round or nearly so in general form; spherical.

INFLORESCENCE: The arrangement or grouping of flowers in a branch system (Figure 55).

LANCEOLATE: Narrow, with widest point near the base and tapering to the apex (Figure 54).

LEAFLET: The bladelike portion of a divided (compound) leaf (Figure 52).

LEGUME: Practically any dry fruit splitting along two lines and having one row of seeds. The fruit type of the bean family.

NARCOTIC: A drug which in moderate doses causes insensibility and relieves pain; in larger doses produces stupor and convulsions.

NAUSEA: Uneasiness of the stomach with a desire to vomit.

NODE: Position on a stem where a leaf is attached (Figure 52).

OPPOSITE: Two leaves, opposing each other, at any one level on a stem; two leaves at a node (Figure 52).

OVARY (of flower): Lower portion of pistil, contains the ovules (Figure 55).

OVATE: Relatively wide and broadest near the base (Figure 54).

OVOID: Egg-shaped, with the greatest diameter near the base.

OVULE: Structure in ovary which contains the egg and which develops into the seed after fertilization of the egg.

PALMATE: Radiating from a common point: palmately veined (Figure 52) or palmately divided leaf (Figure 53).

PANICLE: A rather broad and often many-branched inflorescence (Figure 55).

PERENNIAL: Plants that continue to live year after year.

PERIANTH: Collective term for the sepals and petals of a flower (Figure 55).

PETAL: One unit of the inner whorl of sterile leaflike parts of a flower; usually colored and showy (Figure 55).

PETIOLE: The stalk of a leaf.

PINNATE: Arranged along a central axis; pinnately veined (Figure 52) or pinnately divided leaf (Figure 53).

PISTIL: The central structure(s) of a flower which develops into the fruit after fertilization (Figure 55).

PITH: The soft spongy central cylinder of most stems (Figure 52).

POLLEN: Minute granular structures produced in the anthers of the flower (Figure 55) and necessary for sexual reproduction in seed plants.

POME: A fleshy fruit with a fleshy outer portion and a papery "core"; an apple is a pome.

RACEME: A rather elongated and slender inflorescence in which the pedicels are attached to a simple central axis and are unbranched (Figure 55).

RESPIRATORY: Pertaining to the lungs and other organs for breathing.

RHIZOME: An underground stem, often horizontal.

RING: A thin, loose tissue around the stalk of a mushroom; often called the veil or annulus (Figure 51).

ROOTSTOCK: A rhizome or the perennial source of stems and roots; or used as a general term for any root system.

SALIVATION: An excessive discharge of saliva from the mouth.

SEED: A ripened ovule after fertilization of the egg;

embryonic plant within a protective coat, which will germinate into a new plant.

SEPAL: One unit of the outer whorl of sterile leaflike parts of a flower; often green but sometimes colored (Figure 55).

SIMPLE: A leaf blade which is not divided into leaflets (Figure 53).

SPASM: An uncontrolled and unnatural muscular contraction.

SPIKE: An inflorescence which is generally long, slender and with sessile flowers (Figure 55).

SPORE: A minute structure, not a seed, which is capable of developing into a new individual; a reproductive body in non-seed plants.

STALK: Stemlike structure at the base of a flower or leaf (used here in place of pedicel, peduncle, petiole) (Figure 53).

STAMEN: The part of the flower in which the pollen is produced; the pollen-bearing organ of a flower composed of anther (pollen sac) and filament (stalk) (Figure 55).

STIPULE: One or two small bracts or leaves at the base of a leaf (Figure 53).

STUPOR: Partial or complete unconsciousness.

TREMOR: An involuntary trembling, shivering, or shaking.

TUBER: Swollen and fleshy underground stem (as a potato).

UMBEL: A branched flat-topped cluster of small flowers (Figure 55).

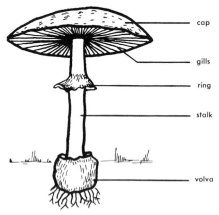

cap

gills

ring

stalk

volva

Figure 51. Parts of a mushroom.

VOLVA: Swollen cup at base of some mushrooms (Figure 51).

WHORLED: Three or more leaves at a node (Figure 52).

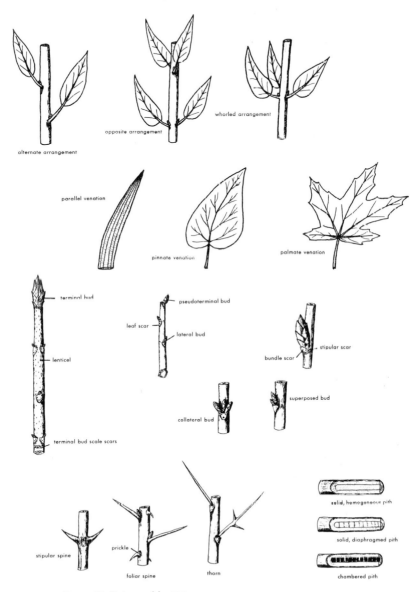

Figure 52. Twigs and leaves.

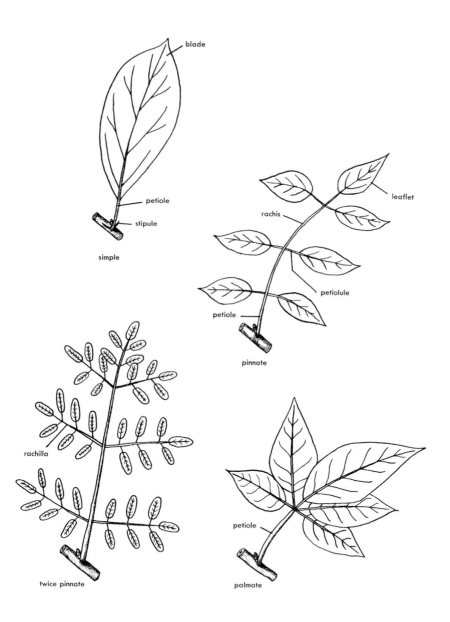

Figure 53. Leaf forms.

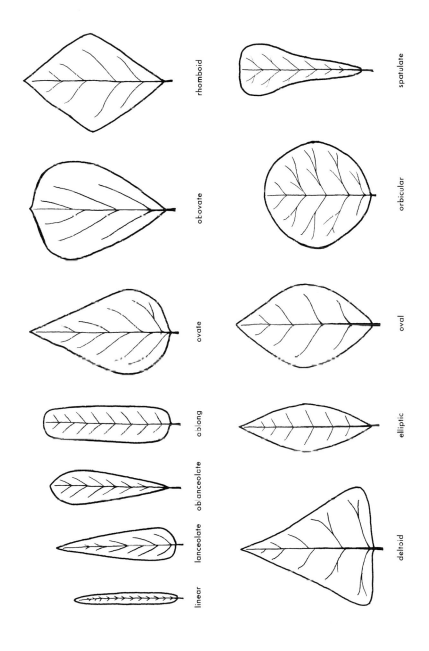

Figure 54. Leaf shapes.

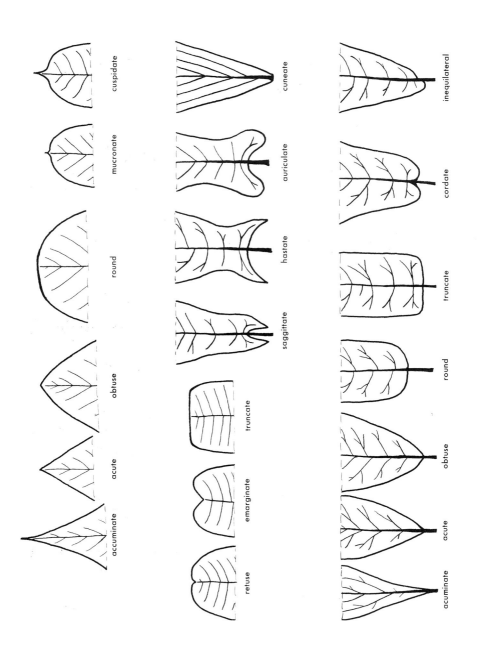

Figure 54. Leaf shapes.

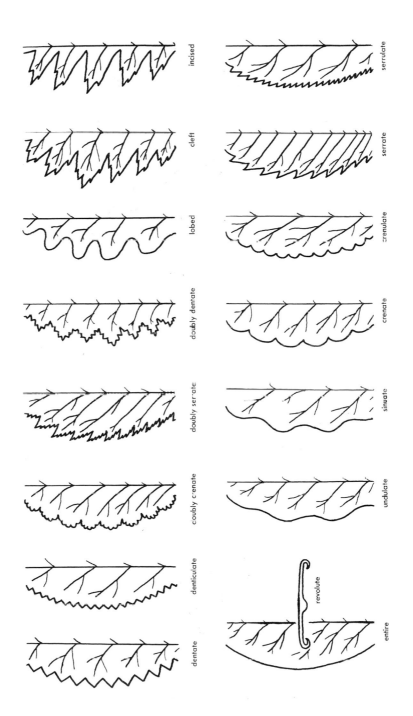

Figure 54. Leaf shapes.

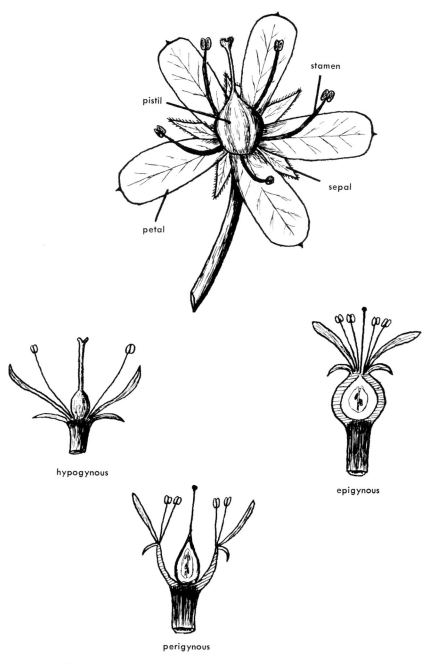

Figure 55. Flower parts and inflorescences.

hypogynous

epigynous

perigynous

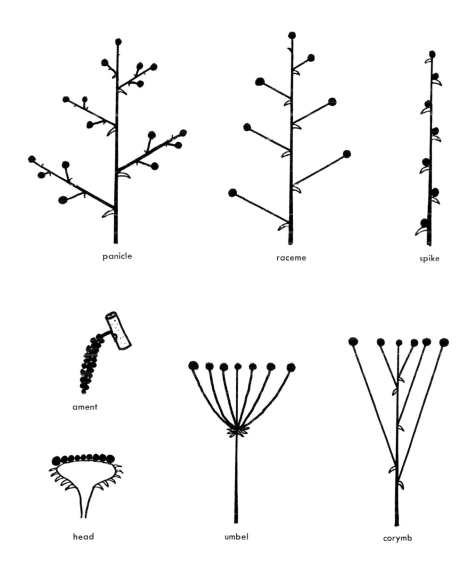

panicle

raceme

spike

ament

head

umbel

corymb

BIBLIOGRAPHY

GENERAL REFERENCES

Arena, Jay M. *Poisoning: Chemistry, Symptoms, Treatments.* Springfield, Ill.: Charles C. Thomas, 1963.

Baskin, Esther. *The Poppy and Other Deadly Plants.* New York: Delacorte Press, 1967.

Deichmann, W. B., and H. W. Gerarde. *Symptomatology and Therapy of Toxicological Emergencies.* New York: Academic Press, 1964.

Duncan, Wilbur H. *Poisonous Plants in the Southeastern United States.* Athens, Ga: the author, 1958.

Fernald, M. L., and A. C. Kinsey. *Edible Wild Plants of Eastern North America* (revised by R. C. Rollins). New York: Harper and Row, 1958.

Gillespie, W. H. *Edible Wild Plants of West Virginia.* New York: Scholar's Library, 1959.

Hardin, James W. *Commercial Herbs, Roots and Pollens of North Carolina.* North Carolina Agricultural Experiment Station Bulletin 435, 1968.

Harrington, H. D. *Edible Native Plants of the Rocky Mountains.* Albuquerque: University of New Mexico Press, 1967.

Harvey, R. B., *et al. Pesky Plants.* University of Minnesota Agricultural Experiment Station Bulletin 381, 1944.

Hesler, L. R. *Mushrooms of the Great Smokies.* Knoxville: University of Tennessee Press, 1960.

Hood, Mary V. *Outdoor Hazards, Real and Fancied.* New York: Macmillan, 1955.

Kingsbury, John M. *Poisonous Plants of the United States and Canada.* Englewood Cliffs, N.J.: Prentice-Hall, 1964.

————. *Deadly Harvest: A Guide to Common Poisonous Plants.* New York: Holt, Rinehart and Winston, 1965.

Lampe, Kenneth F., and Rune Fagerström. *Plant Toxicity and Dermatitis: A Manual for Physicians.* Baltimore: Williams and Wilkins, 1968.

Marderosian, Ara Der. "Poisonous Plants in and around the Home," *American Journal of Pharmaceutical Education,* XXX (1966), 115–140.

Modell, Walter, and Alfred Lansing. *Drugs.* Morristown, N.J.: Silver Burdett, 1967.

Morton, Julia F. "Ornamental Plants with Poisonous Properties," *Proceedings of the Florida State Horticultural Society,* LXXI (1958), 372–380; LXXV (1962), 484–491.

————. *Wild Plants for Survival in South Florida.* Miami: Hurricane House, 1962.

Phillips Petroleum Company. *Pasture and Range Plants, Sec. IV: Poisonous Grassland Plants.* Bartlesville, Okla.: Phillips Petroleum, 1957.

Ramsbottom, J. *Poisonous Fungi.* New York: Penguin Books, 1945.

Sievers, A. F. *American Medicinal Plants of Commercial Importance.* USDA Miscellaneous Publication 77, 1930.

West, Erdman. *Poisonous Plants Around the Home.* Florida Agricultural Experiment Station Circular S-100, 1957.

Wolfe, H. S. *Miscellaneous Tropical and Sub-tropical Florida Fruits.* Florida and USDA Cooperative Extension Bulletin 109, 1941.

Wyeth Laboratories. *The Sinister Garden: A Guide to the Most Common Poisonous Plants.* New York: Wyeth Laboratories, 1966.

POISONOUS PLANT MANUALS, BY STATE AND CANADA

Alabama

Cory, C. A., et al. Poisonous Plants of Alabama. Alabama Polytechnic Institute Extension Circular 71, 1924.

Alaska

Heller, Christine A. Wild Edible and Poisonous Plants of Alaska. University of Alaska and USDA Cooperative Extension Service Bulletin F-40, 1953.

California

Sampson, A. W., and H. E. Malmsten. Stock-poisoning Plants of California. California Agricultural Experiment Station Bulletin 593, 1942.

Canada

Fyles, F. Principal Poisonous Plants of Canada. Canada Department of Agriculture, Dominion Experimental Farms Bulletin 39 (2nd ser.), 1920.

McLean, A., and H. H. Nicholson. Stock Poisoning Plants of the British Columbia Ranges. Canada Department of Agriculture Publication 1037, 1958.

Colorado

Durrell, L. W., et al. Poisonous and Injurious Plants in Colorado. Colorado Agricultural Experiment Station Bulletin 412-A, 1952.

Connecticut

Shepard, C. E., E. M. Bailey, and D. C. Welden. Notes on Livestock Poisoning in Connecticut. Connecticut Agricultural Experiment Station Bulletin 470, 1943.

Florida

Maxwell, Lewis S. Florida's Poisonous Plants, Snakes, Insects. Tampa: L. S. Maxwell, 1963.

West, Erdman, and M. W. Emmel. Poisonous Plants in Florida. Florida Agricultural Experiment Station Bulletin 510, 1952.

Georgia

Duncan, W. H., and T. J. Jones. Poisonous Plants

of Georgia. University of Georgia School of Veterinary Medicine Bulletin XLIX, No. 13, 1949.

Hawaii

Arnold, Harry L. *Poisonous Plants of Hawaii.* Rutland, Vt.: Charles E. Tuttle, 1968.

Idaho

Gail, Floyd W. *Some Poisonous Plants of Idaho.* University of Idaho Agricultural Experiment Station Bulletin 86, 1916.

Illinois

Tehon, L. R., C. C. Morril, and R. Graham. *Illinois Plants Poisonous to Livestock.* Illinois Extension Service Circular 599, 1946.

Indiana

Hansen, A. A. *Indiana Plants Injurious to Livestock.* Purdue Agricultural Experiment Station Circular 175, 1930.

Lee, O. C., and L. P. Doyle. *Indiana Plants Poisonous and Injurious to Livestock.* Purdue Agricultural Extension Service Bulletin 240, 1950.

Kansas

Choguill, H. S. *Some Poisonous Plants of Kansas.* Kansas Academy of Science Transactions 61(1), 1958.

Kentucky

Hyatt, M. T., R. G. Brown, and J. W. Herron. *Some Plants of Kentucky Poisonous to Livestock.* Kentucky Agricultural Extension Service Circular 502, 1953.

Louisiana

Gowanloch, J. N., and C. A. Brown. *Poisonous Snakes, Plants and Black Widow Spider of Louisiana.* New Orleans: Louisiana Department of Conservation, 1943.

Maryland

Brown, R. G. *Plants Poisonous to Livestock.* Maryland Agricultural Extension Service Fact Sheet 91, 1955.

Reynard, G. B., and J. B. S. Norton. *Poisonous Plants of Maryland in Relation to Livestock.* Maryland Agricultural Experiment Station Bulletin A-10, 1942.

Minnesota

Harvey, R. B., *et al. Weeds Poisonous to Livestock.* Minnesota Agricultural Experiment Station Bulletin 388, 1945.

Mississippi

Therell, J. S., and W. R. Thompson. *Poisonous Trees, Bushes and Stumps.* Mississippi Agricultural Extension Service Agronomy Folder 10, 1949.

Montana

Welch, H., and H. E. Morris. *Range Plants Poisonous to Livestock in Montana.* Montana Agricultural Experiment Station Circular 197, 1952.

New Mexico

Hershey, A. L. *Some Poisonous Plant Problems of New Mexico.* New Mexico Agricultural Experiment Station Bulletin 322, 1945.

Norris, J. J., and K. A. Valentine. *Principal Poisonous Plants of New Mexico Ranges.* New Mexico Agricultural Experiment Station Bulletin 390, 1954.

New York

Muenscher, W. C., and W. T. Winne. *Common Poisonous Plants.* Cornell Agricultural Extension Service Bulletin 538, 1955.

North Carolina

Hardin, James W. *Poisonous Plants of North Carolina.* North Carolina Agricultural Experiment Station Bulletin 414, 1961.

————. *Stock-poisoning Plants of North Carolina.* North Carolina Agricultural Experiment Station Bulletin 414 (revised), 1966.

North Dakota

Stevens, O. A. *Poisonous Plants and Plant Products.* North Dakota Agricultural Experiment Station Bulletin 265, 1933.

Ohio

Schaffner, J. H. "Poisonous and Other Injurious Plants of Ohio," *Ohio Naturalist,* IV (1903), 32.

Oklahoma

Featherly, H. I. *Some Plants Poisonous to Livestock*

in Oklahoma. Oklahoma Agricultural Experiment
Station Circular C-118, 1945.

Oregon

Gilkey, H. M. *Livestock-Poisoning Weeds of Oregon.*
Oregon Agricultural Experiment Station Bulletin
564, 1958.

Pennsylvania

Graham, E. H. *Poisonous Plants of Pennsylvania.*
Pittsburgh: Carnegie Museum, 1935.

Gress, E. M. *Poisonous Plants of Pennsylvania.* Pennsylvania Department of Agriculture Bulletin 18(5),
No. 531, 1935.

Texas

Walker, A. H. *Poisonous Range Plants of Texas.* Texas
Agricultural Extension Service Leaflet 114, 1949.

Sperry, O. E., *et al. Texas Range Plants Poisonous to
Livestock.* Texas Agricultural Experiment Station
Bulletin 796, 1955.

Utah

Stoddart, L. A., *et al. Important Poisonous Plants of
Utah.* Utah Agricultural Experiment Station Special
Report 2, 1949.

Virginia

Massey, A. B. *Poisonous Plants.* Virginia Polytechnic
Institute Extension Service Bulletin 222, 1954.

West Virginia

Core, Earl L., *et al. The Poisonous Plants of West
Virginia.* Charleston: West Virginia Department of
Agriculture, 1961.

Wyoming

Beath, O. A., *et al. Poisonous Plants and Livestock
Poisoning.* Wyoming Agricultural Experiment Station
Bulletin 324, 1953.

INDEX TO SCIENTIFIC AND COMMON NAMES

Abrus precatorius, 62
Achras, 127
Aconite, 44
Aconitum, 44
  columbianum, 44
  nepellus, 44
  reclinatum, 44
  uncinatum, 44
Actaea, 44, 127
  alba, 45
  arguta, 45
  pachypoda, 45
  rubra, 45
Adonis, spring, 46
Adonis vernalis, 46
Aesculus, 79
  californica, 79
  glabra, 79
  hippocastanum, 79
  octandra, 79
  parryi, 79
  parviflora, 79
  pavia, 80
  sylvatica, 80
Agave, 12
Agrostemma githago, 54, *55*
Ailanthus altissima, 12
Akebia, 127
Akebia quinata, 127
Akee, 78, 128
Akia, 134
Alder, 9
Aleurites, 127
  fordii, 89
  moluccana, 90
Algae, 9, 28
Allamanda, pink, 109
  purple, 109
  wild, 109
  yellow, 12, 103, *104*
Allamanda cathartica, 12, 103,
  104
Almond, 60
Alocasia, 42
Alsike clover, 15

Amanita, Browning, *31*
Amanita, 31
  brunnescens, 31
  verna, 30
Amaryllidaceae, 39
Amaryllis, 39
Amaryllis family, 39
Ambrosia artemisiifolia, 10, 12
Amelanchier, 127
American beech, 72
Ampelopsis, 127
Anacardium occidentale, 12, 127
Anagallis arvensis, 12
Anemone, 46
Angel's trumpet, 114, *115*
Annona, 127
Anthemis cotula, 12
Anthurium, 42
Apiaceae, 84
Apocynaceae, 103
Apocynum cannabinum, 104, *105*
Apple, 60, 131
  cashew, 127
  crab, 60, 131
  custard, 127
  dog, 128
  gopher, 129
  horse, 14
  kei, 129
  mammee, 131
  may, *47,* 132
  pitch, 129
  pond, 127
  prickly, 130
  seven-year, 128
  squaw, 131
  star, 129
  thorn, 48, *112,* 113
  tiger, 108, 133
  vi, *133*
  wild balsam, 88
Apple cactus, 130
Apple-of-Peru, 116, 131
Apple of Sodom, 120
Aquifoliaceae, 74

Araceae, 40
Aralia, 127
  spinosa, 12, 83
Araliaceae, 83
Arctostaphylos, 127
Ardisia escallonioides, 127
Areca catechu, 42, 128
Areca nut, 42
Arecaceae, 42
Arecastrum romanzoffianum, 128
Argemone mexicana, 48
Arisaema triphyllum, 12, 41, 128
Arnica montana, 124
Arnica root, 124
Aronia, 128
Arrow, green, 131
Arrow arum, 131
Arrowroot, Florida, 34, 134
Arrowwood, 133
Artabotrys uncinatus, 128
Artocarpos, 128
Arum, arrow, 131
Arum family, 40
Asarum canadense, 13
Asclepiadaceae, 109
Asclepias, 109
Ash, 9
  mountain, 133
  poison, 20, 21
Asimina, 128
  triloba, 13
Asparagus, 13, 128
Asparagus officinalis, 13, 128
Aster family, 124
Asteraceae, 124
Atropa belladonna, 111, 128
Autumn crocus, 35
Averrhoa carambola, 128
Avocado, 132
Azalea, 100

Bagpod, 63
Bahama strongbark, 128
Balsam apple, wild, 88
Balsam pear, 88, 131
Banana family, 35
Baneberry, 44, 45, 127
  western, 45
Barbados cherry, 131
Barbados nut, 94, 95
Barberry, 128
Barberry family, 47
Barren strawberry, 134
Bastard toadflax, 129
Bay, California, 133
  red, 132
  sweet, 132
Bean, broad, 68
  castor, 96
  curcas, 94, 95
  English, 68
  fava, 68
  horse, 68

hyacinth, 64
  love, 62
  lucky, 62
  mescal, 68
  prayer, 62
  precatory, 62
  Windsor, 68
Bearberry, 127
Beautybush, 128
Beech, 9, 72
  American, 72
  European, 72
Belamcanda chinensis, 128
Belladonna, 111, 128
Bellyache bush, 94
Benzoin, 130
Berberidaceae, 47
Berberis, 128
Berchemia scandens, 128
Berry, bane, 44, 45
  bear, 127
  black, 132
  blue, 133
  boysen, 132
  buffalo, 133
  bull, 133
  bunch, 129
  China, 77, 78, 131
  choke, 128
  Christmas, 130, 132, 133
  cloud, 132
  coral, 44, 45
  crack, 130
  crow, 130
  curlew, 130
  dew, 132
  dog, 127
  elder, 110, 132
  goose, 132
  hack, 128
  ink, 50, 52
  June, 132
  liver, 133
  locust, 128
  logan, 132
  marl, 127
  nanny, 133
  nagoon, 132
  partridge, 131
  pigeon, 50, 52, 121, 130
  poison, 113
  poke, 50, 52
  salmon, 132
  scoot, 133
  scurvy, 133
  service, 127
  shad, 127
  silver, 130
  snake, 44, 45
  snow, 133
  soap, 133
  sparkle, 133
  squash, 133

sugar, 128
tea, 130
thimble, 132
water, 131
wax, 133
wine, 132
Be-still tree, 108
Betel nut, 42, 128
Birch, 9
Bird-of-paradise, 35, 66
Bird pepper, 13
Bitter gourd, 88
Bittersweet, 128
climbing, 74
European, *119*, 120
Black cherry, 60, *61*
Black gum, 131
Black haw, 128
Black henbane, 114
Black locust, 66, *67*
Black nightshade, 117, *118*
Black sapote, 129
Black snakeroot, 39
Blackberry, 132
Blackberry lily, 128
Bladderpod, 63
Bleeding heart, 13, 50, *51*
Blighia sapida, 78, 128
Blite, strawberry, 129
Bloodroot, 15, 49
Blue cohosh, 13, 48, 128
Blueberry, 133
Bottlebrush buckeye, 79
Bourreria ovata, 128
Bower, virgin's, 13, 46
Box, 58
Box-thorn, 131
Boxwood, 13, 58
Boxwood family, 58
Boysenberry, 132
Brassicaceae, 88
Brazil nut, 73
Brazilian pepper, 15
Breadfruit, 128
Breeches, Dutchman's, 50
Broad bean, 68
Broccoli, 88
Browning amanita, *31*
Brussels sprouts, 88
Buckeye, 79
bottlebrush, 79
California, 79
Ohio, 79
painted, *80*
red, 80
yellow, 79
Buckeye family, 79
Buckthorn, 75, 128, 132
Buckthorn family, 75
Buckwheat family, 58
Buffalo berry, 133
Buffalo nut, 132
Bull nettle, 16

Bullberry, 133
Bumelia, 128
Bunchberry, 129
Burning bush, 23, 74
Burrow weed, 126
Buttercup, 14, 47
Buttercup family, 44
Button, mescal, 56, *57*
Buxaceae, 58
Buxus sempervirens, 13, 58
Byrsonima lucidum, 128

Cabbage, 88
Cabbage palm, 132
Cactaceae, 56
Cactus, apple, 130
opuntia, 131
tree, 128
Cactus family, 56
Cajeput, 14
Caladium, 42
California bay, 133
California buckeye, 79
California laurel, 133
Calla palustris, 128
Calla, wild, 128
Callicarpa americana, 128
Calocarpum sapota, 128
Calophyllum inophyllum, 128
Calotropis gigantea, 109
Caltha palustris, 46
Caltrop family, 83
Camas, death, 39
Campsis radicans, 13, *15*
Cananga odorata, 128
Candlenut, 90, 127
Canistel, 131
Cannabaceae, 70
Cannabis sativa, 70, *71*
Cannonball tree, 73
Caper spurge, 91
Caprifoliaceae, 110
Capsicum frutescens, 13, 128
Carambola, 128
Cardinal flower, 122
Carica papaya, 13, 128
Carrion flower, 133
Carissa, 128
Carissa grandiflora, 128
Carolina jessamine, 102, *103*
Carrot, wild, 13
Carrot family, 84
Caryophyllaceae, 54
Caryota, 128
mitis, 13
Casasia clusiaefolia, 128
Cascara, 132
Cashew apple, 127
Cashew nut, 12
Cassava, 94
Castor bean, *96*
Castor-oil plant, *96*
Catalpa, 13

Cauliflower, 88
Caulophyllum thalictroides, 13,
  48, 128
Cedar, 9, 130
  red, 14
  stinking, 133
Celandine, 13, 49
Celastraceae, 74
Celastrus scandens, 74, 128
Celtis, 128
Century plant, 12
Cephalocereus, 128
Cereus, night-blooming, 130
Ceriman, 131
Cestrum, 113
  green, 113
Cestrum, 129
  diurnum, 113
  nocturnum, 113
  parqui, 113
Chain, golden, 65
Chaenomeles, 129
Chalice vine, 117
Chelidonium majus, 13, 49
Chenopodium capitatum, 129
Cherimoya, 127
Cherry, 60, 132
  Barbados, 131
  black, 60, 61
  finger, 73, 132
  ground, 116, 132
  Jerusalem, 116, 120
  laurel, 60
  Surinam, 130
  wild, 60, 61
Cherry laurel, 60
Chili pepper, 128
Chimaphila umbellata, 13
Chinaball tree, 77, 78
Chinaberry, 77, 78, 131
Chinatree, 77, 78
Chinese lantern, 116
Chionanthus virginicus, 129
Chokeberry, 128
Christmas berry, 130, 132, 133
Christmas rose, 46
Chrysanthemum, 13
Chrysobalanus, 129
Chrysophyllum, 129
Cicuta maculata, 84
Citharexylum fruticosum, 129
Cissus, 127
Citrus, 129
  aurantifolia, 13, 129
  aurantium, 129
  trifoliatus, 129
Clematis, 46
  virginiana, 13
Climbing bittersweet, 74
Climbing lily, 36, 37
Climbing nightshade, 119, 120
Clintonia, 129
Clintonia borealis, 129

Clitocybe, 31
  illudens, 32
Cloudberry, 132
Clover, alsike, 15
Club, Hercules', 12, 83, 127
Clusia rosea, 129
Cnidoscolus, 13
  stimulosus, 16
Coca, 81
Coca family, 81
Coccoloba, 129
Coccothrinax argentata, 129
Cocculus, 129
Cockle, 54, 55
  corn, 54, 55
Coconut palm, 129
Cocoplum, 129
Cocos nucifera, 129
Coffee, wild, 133
Coffee tree, Kentucky, 64
Cohosh, blue, 13, 48, 128
  white, 44, 45
Colchicum autumnale, 35
Colocasia, 42
Comandra, 129
Compositae, 124
Conium maculatum, 13, 86
Convallaria, 36
  majalis, 36
  montana, 36
Coontie, 34, 134
Coralberry, 44, 45
Coral plant, 94
Coral sumac, 18
Cordia, scarlet, 129
Cordia sebestena, 129
Corn, squirrel, 50
  turkey, 50
Corn cockle, 54, 55
Cornus, 129
Cotoneaster, 129
Cowbane, spotted, 84
Cowitch, 13, 15
Cowslip, 130
Coyotillo, 75, 130
Crab apple, 60, 131
Crabseye, 62
Crackberry, 130
Cranberry, 133
Crape jasmine, 106
Crataegus, 129
Creeper, trumpet, 13, 15
  Virginia, 75, 76, 131
Creeping cucumber, 131
Cress, 88
Crinum, 39
Crocus, autumn, 35
Crosier, 34
Crosier cycas, 34
Crowberry, 130
Crowfoot, 47
Crownflower, 109
Crown-of-thorns, 91
Cruciferae, 88

Cryptostegia, 13, 109
  grandiflora, 109
  madagascariensis, 13
Cucumber, creeping, 131
  Indian, 131
  wild, 133
Cucurbitaceae, 88
Curcas bean, 94, 95
Curlewberry, 130
Currant, 132
Custard apple, 127
Cycadaceae, 34
Cycad, 34, 129
Cycas, crosier, 34
Cycas, 34
  circinalis, 34, 129
Cydonia oblonga, 129
Cypress spurge, 90
Cypripedium, 13

Daffodil, 39
Daisy, 13
Daisy fleabane, 13
Daphne, 72, 129
Daphne mezereum, 72, 129
Darling plum, 132
Datura, 112, 113
Datura, 13, 112, 113, 115
  metaloides, 113
  metel, 114
  stramonium, 13, 112, 113
  suaveolens, 114, 115
Daubentonia punicea, 63
Daucus carota, 13
Day-blooming jessamine, 113
Deadly nightshade, 111, 119, 120
Death camas, 39
Delphinium, 46
  ajacis, 13
Destroying angel, 30
Devil's trumpet, 114
Devil's walkingstick, 83
Devilwood, 131
Dewberry, 132
Dewdrop, golden, 121
Dicentra, 13, 50, 51
  eximia, 51
Dictamnus albus, 22
Dieffenbachia, 40
  picta, 40
  seguine, 40
Digitalis purpurea, 121
Dilly, 127
Dinner bell, monkey, 93
Dioon, 34
Diospyros, 129
Diphylleia cymosa, 129
Dirca palustris, 13
Disporum, 129
Dittany, 22, 23
Dock, 15
Dog apple, 128

Dog fennel, 12
Dogbane, 104, 105
Dogbane family, 103
Dogberry, 127
Dogwood, 129
Dolichos lablab, 64
Doll's-eyes, 44, 45
Dovyalis, 129
Downy myrtle, 73, 132
Downy thornapple, 114
Duchesnea indica, 130
Dumbcane, 40
Duranta, 121
Duranta repens, 121, 130
Dutchman's breeches, 50

Eggfruit, 131
Elaeagnus, 130
Elder, 110
  gulf, 111
  Mexican, 111
  poison, 20, 21
  red-berried, 111
  southern, 111
Elderberry, 110, 132
Elephant ears, 42
Elm, 9
Empetrum, 130
English bean, 68
English ivy, 14, 83, 130
Ephedra, 130
Ericaceae, 98
Erigeron canadensis, 13
Ergot, 29, 71
Eriobotrya japonica, 130
Ervatamia coronaria, 106
Erythroxylaceae, 81
Erythroxylon coca, 81
Eugenia, 130
Euonymus, 74, 130
Eupatorium rugosum, 124, 125
Euphorbia, 13, 17, 90
  corollata, 90
  cyparissias, 90
  lathyris, 91
  maculata, 17
  marginata, 91
  milii, 91
  pulcherrima, 92
  splendens, 91
  tirucallii, 92, 93
Euphorbiaceae, 89
European beech, 72
European bittersweet, 119, 120
Everlasting pea, 65
Eyebane, 17

Fabaceae, 62
Fagaceae, 72
Fagus, 72
  grandifolia, 72
  sylvatica, 72
Fall poison, 124, 125

False hellebore, 38
False mastic, 133
False poinciana, 63
False sago palm, 34, 129
False solomon's seal, 133
Fan palm, 134
Fava bean, 68
Feijoa sellowiana, 130
Fern, 34
Fern palm, 34
Feverwort, 133
Ficus, 13, 130
Fiddle, monkey, 92, *93*
Fiddlehead, 34
Fiddlewood, Florida, 129
Fig, 13, 130
Finger cherry, 73, 132
Firecracker plant, 80
Firethorn, 132
Fishtail palm, 128
   tufted, 13
Flacourtia indica, 130
Flag, 14
Flame vine, Mexican, 15
Flax, 131
Fleabane, daisy, 13
Florida arrowroot, 34, 134
Florida fiddlewood, 129
Flower, cardinal, 122
   carrion, 133
   crown, 109
   kahili, 14
   pasque, 46
   sky, 121
   trumpet, 117
   wind, 46
Flowering quince, 129
Flowering spurge, 90
Fool's parsley, poison, *86*
Forestiera, 130
Fortunella, 130
Four-o'clock, 56
Four-o'clock family, 56
Foxglove, 121
Fragaria, 130
Frangipani, 14
Fraxinella, 23
French mulberry, 128
Fringe tree, 129
Fumariaceae, 50
Fumitory family, 50
Fungi, 9, 29

Gas plant, 22, 23
Gaultheria, 130
*Gaylussacia,*130
Geiger tree, 129
Gelsemium, 14, 102, *103*
   rankinii, 102
   sempervirens, 14, 102, *103*
Gentian, horse, 133
Ginger, wild, 13
Ginkgo, 14, 130

Ginkgo biloba, 14, 130
Ginseng, 131
Ginseng family, 83
Gleditsia triacanthos, 65
Gloriosa superba, 36, *37*
Glory lily, 36, *37*
Glottidium, 63
Golden chain, 65
Golden dewdrop, 121
Golden seal, 46
Goldenrod, rayless, 126
Gooseberry, 132
Gooseberry, hill, 73
   otaheite, 132
Gopher apple, 129
Gourd, bitter, 88
Gourd family, 88
Grape, 133
   sea, 129
   shore, 129
Grape family, 75
Grapefruit, 129
Grass, 9
Green arrow, 131
Green cestrum, 113
Greenbriar, 133
Grevillea banksii, 14
Ground cherry, 116, 132
Ground hemlock, 34, 133
Ground oak, 129
Guaiacum officinale, 83
Guarsteen, 130
Guava, 132
   pineapple, 130
Gulf elder, 111
Gum, black, 131
   sour, 131
Gymnocladus dioica, 64

Hackberry, 128
Haplopappus heterophyllus, 126
Harrisia, 130
Hashish, 70, *71*
Haw, 133
Hawthorn, 129
Heart, bleeding, 13, 50, *51*
Hearts-a-bustin', 74
Heath family, 98
Hedera helix, 14, 83, 130
Hedge, 100
Hedysarum mackenzii, 65
Hellebore, 15, 38
   false, 38
Helleborus niger, 46
Hemlock, 88
   ground, 34, 133
   poison, 13, *86*
   spotted water, *84*
   water, *84*
Hemp, 70, *71*
Hemp, Indian, 104, *105*
Hemp family, 70
Henbane, 114

Henbane, black, 114
Hercules' club, 12, 83, 127
Hesperocnide, 14, 22
Heteromeles arbutifolia, 130
Hickory, 9
Hill gooseberry, 73
Hip, rose, 132
Hippeastrum, 39
Hippocastanaceae, 79
Hippomane mancinella, 14, 17, 92, 130
Hobblebush, 133
Hogplum, 133, 134
Holly, 74, 130
  Oregon, 131
Holly family, 74
Honey locust, 64
Honeysuckle, 131
Honeysuckle family, 110
Horse apple, 14
Horse bean, 68
Horse gentian, 133
Horse nettle, 117, *119*
Horsechestnut, 79
Horseradish, 88
Horsesugar, 133
Horseweed, 13
Huckleberry, 130
Hunter's robe, 14
Hura crepitans, 93
Husk tomato, 132
Hyacinth, 38
Hyacinth bean, 64
Hyacinthus orientalis, 38
Hydrangea, 59
  mountain, 59
  oak-leaf, 59
  snowy, 59
Hydrangea, 59
  arborescens, 59
  macrophylla, 59
  quercifolia, 59
  radiata, 59
Hydrastis canadensis, 46
Hylocereus undatus, 130
Hyoscyamus niger, 114
Hypericum perforatum, 14

Ilex, 74, 130
  vomitoria, 74
Indian cucumber, 131
Indian hemp, 104, *105*
Indian jujube, 134
Indian poke, 38
Indian strawberry, 130
Indian tobacco, 14, 122, 124
Indian tree spurge, 92, *93*
Inkberry, 50, *52*
Iris, 14
Irish potato, 120
Ivy, 83
  English, 14, 83, 130
  mountain, 98, *99*
  poison, 15, *19*, 133

Ivy bush, 98, *99*

Jack-in-the-pulpit, 12, *41*, 128
Jack-o'-lantern mushroom, 31, *32*
Jackfruit, 128
Jakfruit, 128
Jamestown weed, *112*, 113
Japan plum, 130
Jasmine, Crape, *106*. See also Jessamine
Jatropha, 94, 130
  curcas, 94, *95*
  gossypifolia, 94
  integerrima, 94
  multifida, 94
  stimulosa, 16
Java plum, 130
Jequirity pea, *62*
Jerusalem cherry, 116, 120
Jessamine, 113, 129. See also Jasmine
  Carolina, 102, *103*
  day-blooming, 113
  night-blooming, 113
  willow-leaved, 113
  yellow, 14, 102, *103*
Jetbead, 60
Jetberry bush, 60
Jimmy weed, 126
Jimsonweed, 13, *112*, 113
Jonquil, 39
Jujube, 134
  Indian, 134
Juneberry, 132
Jungle plum, 133
Juniper, 9, 14, 130
Juniperus, 130
  virginiana, 14

Kahili flower, 14
Kale, 88
Kalmia, 98, *99*
  angustifolia, 98
  latifolia, 98, *99*
  polifolia, 98
Karwinskia humboldtiana, 75, 130
Kei-apple, 129
Kentucky coffee tree, 64
Ketembilla, 129
Key lime, 129
Kinnikinik, 127
Knotweed, 14
Kumquat, 130

Lablab, 64
Laburnum anagyroides, 65
Lactarius, 31
Ladies, naked, 35
Lady's slipper orchid, 13
Lambkill, 98
Lanalana, 128
Langsir, 132

Lantana, 122, *123*, 130
Lantana camara, 122, *123*
Lantern, Chinese, 116
Laportea canadensis, 14, 17
Larkspur, 13, 46
Lathyrus, 65
Laurel, 100, *101*
  California, 133
  cherry, 60
  mountain, 98, *99*
  sheep, 98
  spurge, 72
  swamp, 98
Leaf, satin, 129
  umbrella, 129
Leatherwood, 13
Lecythidaceae, 73
Lecythis family, 73
Leguminosae, 62
Lemon, 129
Leonurus cardiaca, 14
Leopard's-bane, 124
Lepiota, Morgan's, 32, *33*
Lepiota, 32
  molybdites, *33*
Lignum vitae, 83
Ligustrum, 100
Ligustrum, 130
  vulgare, 100
Liliaceae, 35
Lily, blackberry, 128
  climbing, 36, *37*
  glory, 36, *37*
Lily family, 35
Lily-of-the-valley, 36
  wild, 131
Lily turf, 131
Lime, 13, 129
  key, 129
  Spanish, 131
Lindera benzoin, 130
Linum, 131
Liriope, 131
Litchi, 131
Litchi sinensis, 131
Liverberry, 133
Lobelia, 14, 122
Lobelia family, 122
Lobelia inflata, 14, 124
Lobeliaceae, 122
Locust, black, 66, *67*
  honey, 64
Locust berry, 128
Loganberry, 132
Logania family, 102
Loganiaceae, 102
Lonicera, 131
Lophophora williamsii, 56, *57*
Loquat, 130
  Queensland, 73
Loranthaceae, 76
Love bean, *62*
Lucky bean, *62*

Lucky nut, 108
Lucuma nervosa, 131
Lychee, 131
Lycium, 131
Lycopersicon esculentum, 115
LSD, 57, 71

Maclura pomifera, 14
Macrozamia, 34
Mahogany family, 77
Mahonia, 131
Maianthemum canadense, 131
Maidenhair tree, 14, 130
Malabar tree, 92, *93*
Malpighia glabra, 131
Malus, 60, 131
Mamey, 131
Mammea americana, 131
Mammee apple, 131
Mamoncillo, 131
Manchineel, 14, 17, 92, 130
Mandarin, 133
  yellow, 129
Mandrake, 14, *47*, 132
Mangifera indica, 14, 131
Mango, 14, 131
Manihot esculenta, 94
Manioc, 94
Manzanita, 127
Maple, 9
Marigold, marsh, 46
Marihuana, 70, *71*
Marijuana, 58, 70, *71*
Marlberry, 127
Marsh marigold, 46
Marvel-of-Peru, 56
Mastic, false, 133
Mast-wood, 128
Matrimony vine, 131
Mayapple, 14, *47*, 132
Maypop, 131
Meadow saffron, 35
Medeola virginiana, 131
Melaleuca leucadendra, 14
Melia azedarach, 77, *78*, 131
Meliaceae, 77
Melicocca bijuga, 131
Melonette, 131
Melothria pendula, 131
Menispermaceae, 43
Menispermum canadense, *43*, 131
Mescal, 56, *57*
Mescal bean, 68
Mescal button, 56, *57*
Metel, 114
Metopium toxiferum, 14, 18, 131
Mexican elder, 111
Mexican flame vine, 15
Mexican pricklepoppy, 48
Mezereum family, 72
Microcycas, 34
Milk bush, 92, *93*
Milk purslane, 17

Milkweed, 109
Milkweed family, 109
Milky-cap mushroom, 31
Mirabilis jalapa, 56
Mistletoe, 27, 76, *77*, 132
Mistletoe family, 76
Mitchella repens,131
Mole plant, 91
Momordica charantia, 88, 131
Monkey dinner bell, 93
Monkey fiddle, 92, 93
Monkey pot, 73
Monkshood, 44
Monstera, 42, 131
Monstera deliciosa, 131
Moonseed, *43*, 129, 131
Moonseed family, 43
Moraceae, 70
Morel, 30
Morgan's lepiota, 32, *33*
Morning glory, 71
Morus, 131
  alba, 70
  rubra, 14, 70
Motherwort, 14
Mountain ash, 133
Montain hydrangea, 59
Mountain ivy, 98, *99*
Mountain laurel, 98, *99*
Mountain snuff, 124
Mountain tobacco, 124
Moxieplum, 130
Mulberry, 131
  French, 128
  red, 14, 70
  white, 70
Mulberry family, 70
Musaceae, 35
Mushroom, 29
Mustard, 88
Mustard family, 88
Myristica fragrans, 42
Myristicaceae, 42
Myrtaceae, 73
Myrtle, 131
  downy, 73, 132
Myrtle family, 73
Myrtus communis, 131

Nagoonberry, 132
Naked ladies, 35
Nandina, 131
Nandina domestica, 131
Nannyberry, 133
Narcissus, 39
Natal plum, 128
Nerium, 14, *107*, 108
  indicum, 108
  oleander, 14, *107*
Nettle, 17
  bull, 16
  horse, 117, *119*
  spurge, 13, 16

stinging, 15, 22, *23*
  western stinging, 14
  wood, 14, 17
Nicandra physalodes, 116, 131
Nicotiana, 116
  glauca, 116
  tabacum, 116
  trigonophylla, 116
Night-blooming cereus, 130
Night-blooming jessamine, 113
Nightshade, 117, 133
  black, 117, *118*
  climbing, *119*, 120
  deadly, 111, *119*, 120
  yellow, 109
Nut, areca, 42
  Barbados, 94, *95*
  betel, 42, 128
  buffalo, 132
  candle, 90, 127
  cashew, 12
  lucky, 108
  physic, 94, *95*
  purge, 94, *95*, 130
  tung, *89*, 127
Nutmeg, 42
Nutmeg family, 42
Nyctaginaceae, 56
Nyssa, 131

Oak, 9, 72
  ground, 129
  poison, 15, 19, 133
  western poison, 18
Oak family, 72
Oak leaf hydrangea, 59
Ochrosia elliptica, 108, 131
Ochrosia plum, 108, 131
Ohio buckeye, 79
Old man's beard, 129
Oleaceae, 100
Oleander, 14, *107*
  yellow, 108
Oleaster, 130
Olive, Russian, 130
  wild, 130
Olive family, 100
Olive plum, 129
Opium poppy, 49
Opuntia, 131
Opuntia cactus, 131
Orange, 129
  Osage, 14
  Seville, 129
  sour, 129
  trifoliate, 129, 132
Orchid, lady's slipper, 13
Oregon holly, 131
Ornithogalum umbellatum, 38
Osage orange, 14
Osmanthus, 131
Otaheite gooseberry, 132
Oyster plant, 15

Painted buckeye, *80*
Palm, betel nut, 42
  cabbage, 132
  coconut, 129
  false sago, 34, 129
  fan, 134
  fern, 34
  palmetto, 132
  royal, 132
  silver, 129
  thatch, 129
  tufted fishtail, 13
  Washington, 134
Palm family, 42
Palmae, 42
Palmetto, saw, 133
Palmetto palm, 132
Panax quinquefolia, 131
Papaver somniferum, 49
Papaveraceae, 48
Papaya, 13, 128
Paradise tree, 133
Parilla, yellow, *43*
Parsley, poison fool's, *86*
Parsnip, wild, 22, 23
Parthenocissus, 75, 76, 131
  quinquefolia, 75, 76, 131
  vitacea, 75
Partridgeberry, 131
Pasqueflower, 46
Passiflora, 131
Passion fruit, 131
Pastinaca sativa, 22
Pawpaw, 13, 128
Pea, everlasting, 65
  jequirity, *62*
  rosary, *62*
  singletary, 65
  sweet, 65
  wild sweet, 65
Pea family, 62
Peach, 60, 132
Pear, 132
  balsam, 88, 131
  prickly, 131
Peltandra virginica, 131
Pencil tree, 13, 92, *93*
Pepper, bird, 13
  Brazilian, 15
  chili, 128
Peraphyllum ramosissimum, 131
Peregrina, 94
Persea, 132
  americana, 132
  borbonia, 132
Persimmon, 129
Peru, apple-of-, 116, 131
  marvel-of-, 56
Peyote, 56, *57*
Phacelia, 14
Pheasant's eye, 46

Philodendron, 42
Phoradendron, 27, 76, 77, 132
  flavescens, 27, 76, 77
  serotinum, 27, 76, 77, 132
Photinia, 132
Phyllanthus acidus, 132
Physalis, 116, 132
  peruviana, 117
Physic nut, 94, *95*
Phytolacca, 132
  americana, 50, *53*
  rigida, 50, *53*, 54
Phytolaccaceae, 50
Pickerelweed, 132
Pigeon plum, 129
Pigeonberry, 50, *52*, 121, 130
Pikeweed, 132
Pimpernel, scarlet, 12
Pine, prince's, 13
Pineapple-guava, 130
Pink allamanda, 109
Pink family, 54
Pipsissewa, 13
Pitaya, 130
Pitch apple, 129
Pithecellobium, 14
Pithecellobium dulce, 14
Plum, 60, 132
  coco, 129
  darling, 132
  hog, 133, 134
  Japan, 130
  java, 130
  jungle, 133
  moxie, 130
  natal, 128
  ochrosia, 108, 131
  olive, 129
  pigeon, 129
  saffron, 178
  tallowwood, 134
Plumbago, 14
Plumbago capensis, 14
Plumeria, 14
Podophyllum peltatum, 14, *47*,
  132
Poinciana, 66
  false, 63
Poinciana gilliesii, 66
Poinsettia, 13, 17, 92
Poison, fall, 124, *125*
Poison ash, 20, *21*
Poison elder, 20, *21*
Poison fool's parsley, *86*
Poison hemlock, 13, *86*
Poison ivy, 15, *19*, 133
Poison oak, 15, 19, 133
Poison oak, western, 18
Poison sumac, 15, 20, *21*, 133
Poison wood, 14, 18, 131
Poisonberry, 113
Poke, 50, *52*
  Indian, 38

Pokeberry, 50, *52*, 132
Pokeweed, 50, *52*
Pokeweed family, 50
Polygonaceae, 58
Polygonatum, 132
Polygonum, 14
Polyscias, 14
Pomegranate, 132
Pometia pinnata,132
Poncirus trifoliata, 132
Pond apple, 127
Pongam, 66
Pongamia pinnata, 66
Pontederia cordata, 132
Poplar, 9
Popolo, yellow-fruited, 120
Poppy, common, 49
   Mexican prickle, 48
   opium, 49
   prickly, 48
   rock, 49
Poppy family, 48
Pot, 70, *71*
Potato, 120
   Irish, 120
   white, 120
Potato family, 111
Prayer bean, *62*
Precatory bean, *62*
Pricklepoppy, Mexican, 48
Prickly apple, 130
Prickly pear, 131
Prickly poppy, 48
Primrose, 14
Primula, 14
Prince's pine, 13
Privet, 100, 130
Prunus, 132
   serotina, 60, *61*
Psidium guajava, 132
Puffball, 30
Punica granatum, 132
Punk tree, 14
Purge nut, 94, *95*, 130
Purple allamanda, 109
Purple queen, 15
Purple sesban, 63
Purslane, milk, 17
Pyracantha, 132
Pyrularia pubera, 132
Pyrus, 132

Queen, purple, 15
Queen palm, 128
Queensland loquat, 73
Quercus, 72
Quince, 129
   flowering, 129

Radish, 88
   horse, 88
Ragweed, *10*, 12
Raisin, wild, 133
Ramontchi, 130

Ranunculaceae, 44
Ranunculus, 14, 47
Raspberry, 132
Rattlebox, 63
Rayless goldenrod, 126
Red bay, 132
Red buckeye, 80
Red cedar, 14
Red mulberry, 14, 70
Red sage, 122, *123*
Red sapote, 128
Red-berried elder, 111
Reynosia septentrionalis, 132
Rhacoma, 132
Rhamnaceae, 75
Rhamnus, 75, 132
   cathartica, 75
   purshiana, 75
Rhaphidophora aurea, 14
Rheum rhaponticum, 58
Rhododendron, 100, *101*
Rhododendron, 100, *101*
   macrophyllum, 100
   maximum, 100, *101*
Rhodomyrtus, 132
   macrocarpa, 73
   tomentosa, 73
Rhodotypos tetrapetala, 60
Rhoeo spathacea, 15
Rhubarb, 58
Rhus, 132
   diversiloba, 18
   radicans, *19*, 20
   toxicodendron, 19
   vernix, 20, *21*
Ribes, 132
Ricinus communis, 96
Rivina humilis, 132
Robinia pseudoacacia, 66, *67*
Robe, hunter's, 14
Rock poppy, 49
Root, arnica, 124
Rosa, 132
Rosaceae, 60
Rosary pea, *62*
Rose, 132
Rose bay, 100, *101*
Rose, Christmas, 46
Rose family, 60
Rose hip, 132
Rouge plant, 132
Royal palm, 132
Roystonea, 132
Rubber vine, 13, 109
Rubus, 132
Rumex, 15
Russian olive, 130
Russula, 32
Rutabaga, 88

Sabal palmetto, 132
Saffron, meadow, 35
Saffron plum, 128
Sage, red, 122, *123*

Sago palm, false, 34, 129
St. John's wort, 14
Salal, 130
Salmonberry, 132
Sambucus, 110, 132
   canadensis, 110, 132
   mexicana, 111
   pubens, 111
   simpsonii, 111
Sandbox tree, 93
Sanguinaria canadensis, 15, 49
Sapindaceae, 78
Sapindus, 133
Sapodilla, 127
Sapote, black, 129
   red, 128
Sarsaparilla, 127
Sassafras, 133
Sassafras albidum, 133
Sassy jack, 91
Satin leaf, 129
Saw palmetto, 133
Saxifragaceae, 59
Saxifrage family, 59
Scarlet cordia, 129
Scarlet pimpernel, 12
Schinus terebinthifolius, 15, 133
Scootberry, 133
Scrophulariaceae, 121
Scurvyberry, 133
Sea grape, 129
Seal, golden, 46
Senecio confusus, 15
Serenoa repens, 133
Serviceberry, 127
Sesban, 63
   purple, 63
Sesbania, 63
Setcreasea purpurea, 15
Seven-year apple, 128
Sevenbark, 59
Seville orange, 129
Shadberry, 127
Sheep laurel, 98
Shepherdia, 133
Shoofly plant, 116
Shore grape, 129
Sideroxylon foetidissimum, 133
Silver leaf, 59
Silver palm, 129
Silverberry, 130
Simarouba glauca, 133
Singletary pea, 65
Skyflower, 121
Smartweed, 14
Smilacina racemosa, 133
Smilax, 133
Snakeberry, 44, 45
Snakeroot, black, 39
   white, 124, *125*
Snapdragon family, 121
Snowberry, 133
Snowdrop, 38
Snow-on-the-mountain, 91

Snowy hydrangea, 59
Snuff, mountain, 124
Soapberry, 133
Soapberry family, 78
Sodom, apple of, 120
Soil algae, 9
Solanaceae, 111
Solandra, 117
Solanum, 117, 133
   americanum, 117, *118*
   carolinense, 117, *119*
   dulcamara, 119, 120
   nigrum, 117
   pseudocapsicum, 120
   sodomeum, 120
   tuberosum, 120
Solomon's seal, 132
   false, 133
Sophora secundiflora, 68
Sorbus, 133
Sorrel, 15
Sour gum, 131
Sour orange, 129
Soursop, 127
Southern elder, 111
Spanish lime, 131
Sparkleberry, 133
Spicebush, 130
Spikenard, 127
Spindle tree, 74
Spondias, 133
Spotted cowbane, *84*
Spotted spurge, 17
Spotted water hemlock, *84*
Spring adonis, 46
Spurge, 13, 90
   caper, 91
   cypress, 90
   flowering, 90
   Indian tree, 92, *93*
   spotted, 17
   stinging, 13, 16
Spurge family, 89
Spurge laurel, 72
Spurge nettle, 13, *16*
Squashberry, 133
Squaw apple, 131
Squirrel corn, 50
Staff-tree family, 74
Staggerweed, 46
Stalk, twisted, 133
Star apple, 129
Star-of-Bethlehem, 38
Stinging nettle, 15, 22, *23*
   western, 14
Stinging spurge, 13, 16
Stinking cedar, 133
Stinkweed, *112,* 113
Stock, 88
Stopper, white, 130
Strawberry, 130
   barren, 134
   Indian, 130
Strawberry blite, 129

Strawberry bush, 74, 130
Strawberry tomato, 116
Strelitzia, 35
Streptopus, 133
Strongbark, 128
  Bahama, 128
Strychnine, 102, 133
Strychnos nux-vomica, 102, 133
Sugarberry, 128
Sumac, 132
Sumac, coral, 18
  poison, 15, 20, *21*, 133
  swamp, 20, *21*
Supplejack, 128
Surinam cherry, 130
Swamp laurel, 98
Swamp sumac, 20, *21*
Sweet pea, 65
Sweetbay, 132
Sweetleaf, 133
Sweetsop, 127
Sycamore, 9
Symphoricarpos, 133
Symplocos tinctoria, 133

Tallowwood plum, 134
Tapioca, 94
Taxaceae, 34
Taxus, 34, 133
  baccata, 34
  brevifolia, 35
  canadensis, 34
  cuspidata, 34
  floridana, 35
Teaberry, 130
Thatch palm, 129
Thevetia peruviana, 108, 133
Thimbleberry, 132
Thimbleweed, 46
Thorn, box-, 131
Thornapple, 48, *112*, 113
Thornapple, downy, 114
Thunderwood, 20, 21
Thymelaeaceae, 72
Tiger apple, 108, 133
Tinker's weed, 133
Toadflax, bastard, 129
Toadstool, 29
Tobacco, 116
  Indian, 14, 122, 124
  mountain, 124
  tree, 116
  wild, 116
Tomato, 115
  husk, 132
  strawberry, 116
  wild, 117, *119*
Torreya, 133
Toxicodendron, 15, 133
  diversilobum, 18
  quercifolium, 19
  radicans, 19
  vernix, 20, *21*
Tread-softly, 16

Tree cactus, 128
Tree spurge, Indian, 92, *93*
Tree tobacco, 116
Tree-of-heaven, 12
Trifoliate orange, 129, 132
Trifolium hybridum, 15
Trillium, 133
Triosteum, 133
Trumpet, angel's, 114, *115*
  devil's, 114
Trumpet creeper, 13, *15*
Trumpet flower, 117
Tufted fishtail palm, 13
Tung nut, *89*, 127
Tung oil tree, *89*
Tupelo, 131
Turf, lily, 131
Turkey corn, 50
Turnip, 88
Twisted stalk, 133

Umbelliferae, 84
Umbellularia californica, 133
Umbrella leaf, 129
Urechites, 109
Urtica dioica, 15, 22, *23*

Vaccinium, 133
Veratrum, 15
  californicum, 38
  parviflorum, 38
  viride, 38
Verbenaceae, 121
Vervain family, 121
Vetchlings, 65
Vi apple, 133
Viburnum, 133
Vicia faba, 68
Virginia creeper, 75, *76*, 131
Virgin's bower, 13, 46
Viscaceae, 76
Vitaceae, 75
Vitis, 133

Wahoo, 74
Wake-robin, 133
Waldsteinia fragarioides, 134
Walkingstick, devil's, 83
Wartweed, 17
Washington palm, 134
Washingtonia filifera, 134
Water hemlock, *84*
Water hemlock, spotted, *84*
Waterberry, 131
Waxberry, 133
Weed, burrow, 126
  Jamestown, *112*, 113
  jimmy, 126
  jimson, *112*, 113
  pickerel, 132
  pike, 132
  poke, 50
  tinker's, 133
Western poison oak, 18

Western stinging nettle, 14
White cohosh, 44, *45*
White mulberry, 70
White potato, 120
White snakeroot, 124, *125*
White stopper, 130
Wi tree, 133
Wicky, 98
Wikstroemia, 134
Wild allamanda, 109
Wild balsam apple, 88
Wild calla, 128
Wild carrot, 13
Wild cherry, 60, *61*
Wild coffee, 133
Wild cucumber, 133
Wild ginger, 13
Wild lily-of-the-valley, 131
Wild olive, 130
Wild parsnip, 22, 23
Wild raisin, 133
Wild sweet pea, 65
Wild tobacco, 116
Wild tomato, 117, *119*
Willow-leafed jessamine, 113
Windflower, 46
Windsor bean, 68
Wineberry, 132
Wintergreen, 130
Wisteria, 69
  sinensis, 69
Wood nettle, 14, 17
Wolfsbane, 44

Ximenia americana, 134

Yellow allamanda, 12, 103, *104*
Yellow buckeye, 79
Yellow jessamine, 14, 102, *103*
Yellow mandarin, 129
Yellow nightshade, 109
Yellow oleander, 108
Yellow parilla, *43*
Yellow-fruited popolo, 120
Yew, 34, 133
Yew family, 34
Ylang-ylang, 128

Zamia, 34, 134
Zigadenus, 39
Zizyphus, 134
  jujuba, 134
  mauritiana, 134
Zygophyllaceae, 83

Réseau de bibliothèques Université d'Ottawa Échéance	Library Network University of Ottawa Date Due